Ambulation in Adults with Central Neurologic Disorders

Editor

FRANCOIS BETHOUX

PHYSICAL MEDICINE AND REHABILITATION CLINICS OF NORTH AMERICA

www.pmr.theclinics.com

Consulting Editor
GREGORY T. CARTER

May 2013 • Volume 24 • Number 2

ELSEVIER

1600 John F. Kennedy Boulevard • Suite 1800 • Philadelphia, Pennsylvania, 19103-2899

http://www.theclinics.com

PHYSICAL MEDICINE AND REHABILITATION CLINICS OF NORTH AMERICA Volume 24, Number 2
May 2013 ISSN 1047-9651, ISBN-978-1-4557-7140-0

Editor: Jessica McCool

Reprints. For copies of 100 or more of articles in this publication, please contact the Commercial Reprints Department, Elsevier Inc., 360 Park Avenue South, New York, NY 10010-1710. Tel.: 212-633-3812; Fax: 212-462-1935; E-mail: reprints@elsevier.com.

Physical Medicine and Rehabilitation Clinics of North America (ISSN 1047-9651) is published quarterly by Elsevier Inc., 360 Park Avenue South, New York, NY 10010-1710. Months of issue are February, May, August, and November. Business and Editorial Offices: 1600 John F. Kennedy Blvd., Suite 1800, Philadelphia, PA 19103-2899. Customer Service Office: 3251 Riverport Lane, Maryland Heights, MO 63043. Periodicals postage paid at New York, NY and additional mailing offices. Subscription price per year is $263.00 (US individuals), $459.00 (US institutions), $140.00 (US students), $320.00 (Canadian individuals), $598.00 (Canadian institutions), $200.00 (Canadian students), $395.00 (foreign individuals), $598.00 (foreign institutions), and $200.00 (foreign students). Foreign air speed delivery is included in all *Clinics* subscription prices. All prices are subject to change without notice. **POSTMASTER:** Send address changes to *Physical Medicine and Rehabilitation Clinics of North America*, Customer Service Office: Elsevier Health Sciences Division, Subscription Customer Service, 3251 Riverport Lane, Maryland Heights, MO 63043. **Customer Service: 1-800-654-2452 (US). From outside of the United States, call 314-447-8871. Fax: 314-447-8029. E-mail: JournalsCustomer Service-usa@elsevier.com (for print support); JournalsOnlineSupport-usa@elsevier.com (for online support).**

Physical Medicine and Rehabilitation Clinics of North America is indexed in *Excerpta Medica, MEDLINE/ PubMed (Index Medicus), Cinahl,* and *Cumulative Index to Nursing and Allied Health Literature.*

Printed and bound by CPI Group (UK) Ltd, Croydon, CR0 4YY

Transferred to digital print 2013

Contributors

CONSULTING EDITOR

GREGORY T. CARTER, MD, MS
Medical Director, Muscular Dystrophy Association Regional Neuromuscular Center, Providence Medical Group, Department of Clinical Neurosciences; Physical Medicine and Rehabilitation Division, Olympia, Washington

EDITOR

FRANCOIS BETHOUX, MD
Director, Rehabilitation Services, The Mellen Center for Multiple Sclerosis Treatment and Research, The Cleveland Clinic Foundation, Cleveland, Ohio

AUTHORS

SHINICHI AMANO, BS
Department of Applied Physiology and Kinesiology, College of Health and Human Performance, University of Florida, Gainesville, Florida

FRANCOIS BETHOUX, MD
Director, Rehabilitation Services, The Mellen Center for Multiple Sclerosis Treatment and Research, The Cleveland Clinic Foundation, Cleveland, Ohio

MARTINA BETSCHART, PT, MSc
Pathokinesiology Laboratory, Centre for Interdisciplinary Research in Rehabilitation of Greater Montreal (CRIR), Institut de réadaptation Gingras-Lindsay-de-Montréal and School of Rehabilitation, University of Montreal, Montreal; The Multidisciplinary SensoriMotor Rehabilitation Research Team, Quebec, Canada

MICHELLE H. CAMERON, MD, PT
Assistant Professor, Department of Neurology, Oregon Health and Science University; Portland VA Medical Center, Portland, Oregon

JOHN CHAE, MD
Professor, Department of Physical Medicine and Rehabilitation, MetroHealth Medical Center, Cleveland Functional Electrical Stimulation Center; Department of Biomedical Engineering, Case Western Reserve University, Cleveland, Ohio

JOAN E. EDELSTEIN, MA, PT, FISPO, CPed
Special Lecturer, Program in Physical Therapy, College of Physicians and Surgeons, Columbia University, New York, New York

ALBERTO ESQUENAZI, MD
John Otto Haas Chair and Professor of PMR and Director MossRehab Gait and Motion Analysis Laboratory, Elkins Park, Pennsylvania

ELIZABETH C. HARDIN, PhD
Principal Investigator, Motion Study Laboratory, Louis Stokes Cleveland VA Medical Center; Research Assistant Professor, Department of Biomedical Engineering, Case Western Reserve University, Cleveland, Ohio

CHRIS J. HASS, PhD
Department of Applied Physiology and Kinesiology, College of Health and Human Performance, University of Florida, Gainesville, Florida

AUDREY L. HICKS, PhD
Department of Kinesiology, McMaster University, Hamilton, Ontario, Canada

RUDI KOBETIC, MSBE
Principal Investigator, Motion Study Laboratory, Louis Stokes Cleveland VA Medical Center, Cleveland, Ohio

ROBERT W. MOTL, PhD
Department of Kinesiology and Community Health, University of Illinois at Urbana-Champaign, Urbana, Illinois

SYLVIE NADEAU, PT, PhD
Pathokinesiology Laboratory, Centre for Interdisciplinary Research in Rehabilitation of Greater Montreal (CRIR), Institut de réadaptation Gingras-Lindsay-de-Montréal and School of Rehabilitation, University of Montreal, Montreal; The Multidisciplinary SensoriMotor Rehabilitation Research Team, Quebec, Canada

YLVA E. NILSAGÅRD, PT, PhD
Centre for Health Care Sciences, Örebro County Council; School of Health and Medical Sciences, Örebro University, Örebro, Sweden

KAREN J. NOLAN, PhD
Research Scientist, Human Performance and Engineering Laboratory, Kessler Foundation Research Center, West Orange; Assistant Professor, Department of Physical Medicine and Rehabilitation, University of Medicine and Dentistry of New Jersey - New Jersey Medical School, Newark, New Jersey

LARA A. PILUTTI, PhD
Department of Kinesiology and Community Health, University of Illinois at Urbana-Champaign, Urbana, Illinois

ARVIND RAMANUJAM, MS
Biomedical Engineer, Human Performance and Engineering Laboratory, Kessler Foundation Research Center, West Orange, New Jersey

RYAN T. ROEMMICH, BS
Department of Applied Physiology and Kinesiology, College of Health and Human Performance, University of Florida, Gainesville, Florida

LYNNE R. SHEFFLER, MD
Assistant Professor, Department of Physical Medicine and Rehabilitation, MetroHealth Medical Center, Cleveland Functional Electrical Stimulation Center, Case Western Reserve University, Cleveland, Ohio

JARED W. SKINNER, MS
Department of Applied Physiology and Kinesiology, College of Health and Human Performance, University of Florida, Gainesville, Florida

RONALD J. TRIOLO, PhD
Executive Director, Motion Study Laboratory, VA Advanced Platform Technology Center, Louis Stokes Cleveland VA Medical Center; Professor, Departments of Orthopaedics and Biomedical Engineering, Case Western Reserve University, Cleveland, Ohio

THEERA VACHRANUKUNKIET, MD
MossRehab Gait and Motion Analysis Laboratory, Elkins Park, Pennsylvania

MATHEW YAROSSI, MS
Biomedical Engineer, Human Performance and Engineering Laboratory, Kessler Foundation Research Center, West Orange; Graduate School of Biomedical Sciences, University of Medicine and Dentistry of New Jersey - New Jersey Medical School, Newark, New Jersey

Contents

Ambulation requires significant motor coordination. Because of inherent differences in body proportions, level of coordination, motivation, and other factors, each individual gait pattern is unique. However, despite the existence of these individual differences that contribute to each person's own unique walking style, there are highly repeatable gait sequences, allowing characterization of normal gait patterns and identification of gait disturbance. This article briefly reviews neural control of human ambulation, basic kinematics, and kinetics of normal human gait, and describes the pathophysiology and clinical presentations of spastic hemiparetic and paraparetic, ataxic, and Parkinsonian gait patterns.

This review discusses challenges faced by clinicians and researchers when measuring ambulation in individuals with central neurologic disorders within 3 distinct environments: clinical, laboratory, and community. Even the most robust measure of ambulation is affected by the environment in which it is implemented and by the clinical or research question and the specificity of the hypothesis being investigated. The ability to accurately measure ambulation (one of the most important metrics used to show transition into a community environment) is essential to measure treatment effectiveness and rehabilitation outcomes in populations with central neurologic disorders.

Many stroke survivors have walking limitations. The results of gait training in individuals who have had strokes are characterized by large confidence intervals for mean differences in gait parameters. An individualized approach to therapy is needed, based on personalized gait pattern indicators and sensorimotor impairments. Three-dimensional gait analysis can help clinicians design the best locomotor training strategy for their patients, and can determine whether a patient is responding to the chosen intervention. Spatiotemporal parameters allow the characterization of the gait of hemiparetic patients but, used alone, they do not allow the cause of the deviations to be inferred.

ubiquitous and life-altering consequences, underscoring the importance of continued efforts to identify approaches to prevent and forestall this event, and to restore walking ability in persons with MS.

Many people with multiple sclerosis MS (PwMS) have impaired balance and walking, and fall frequently. High-quality measures of imbalance and fall risk are essential for identifying who may benefit from interventions to improve balance and prevent falls, and for selecting the most appropriate interventions. We recommend the International Classification of Functioning, Disability and Health (ICF) model. Many measures are available to assess factors affecting balance, fall risk, and walking at the different levels of the ICF. Combining these measures provides the most complete assessment of the individual and the best guidance for interventions by the health care team.

Walking is possible for many patients with a spinal cord injury. Avenues enabling walking include braces, robotics and FES. Among the benefits are improved musculoskeletal and mental health, however unrealistic expectations may lead to negative changes in quality of life. Use rigorous assessment standards to gauge the improvement of walking during the rehabilitation process, but also yearly. Continued walking after discharge may be limited by challenges, such as lack of accessibility in and outside the home, and complications, such as shoulder pain or injuries from falls. It is critical to determine the risks and benefits of walking for each patient.

Parkinson disease is a progressive neurodegenerative disorder characterized by a variety of motor and nonmotor features. This article reviews the problems of postural instability and gait disturbance in persons with Parkinson disease through the discussion of (1) the neuropathology of parkinsonian motor deficits, (2) behavioral manifestations of gait and postural abnormalities observed in persons with Parkinson disease, and (3) pharmacologic, surgical, and physical therapy–based interventions to combat postural instability and gait disturbance. This article advances the treatment of postural instability and gait disturbance by condensing up-to-date knowledge and making it available to clinicians and rehabilitation professionals.

PHYSICAL MEDICINE & REHABILITATION CLINICS OF NORTH AMERICA

RELATED INTEREST

Clinics in Podiatric Medicine and Surgery, April 2012 (Vol. 29, Issue 2)
Foot and Ankle Trauma
Denise M. Mandi, DPM, *Editor*
http://www.podiatric.theclinics.com/

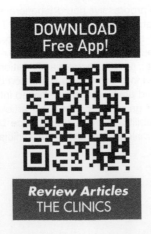

DOWNLOAD Free App!

Review Articles
THE CLINICS

NOW AVAILABLE FOR YOUR iPhone and iPad

Foreword
Ambulation in Adults with Central Neurologic Disorders

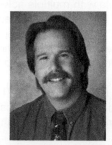

Gregory T. Carter, MD, MS
Consulting Editor

The quality of any body of work is often directly correlated with the strength and vision of the leader of the group. This volume of *Physical Medicine and Rehabilitation Clinics of North America* is no exception. Our editor is Francois Bethoux, MD. Dr Bethoux is an internationally recognized expert in the rehabilitation of patients with complex disorders of the central nervous system (CNS). His research interests include outcomes measurements, including analysis of gait and spasticity in disorders of the CNS. He brings a wealth of knowledge and experience to this project and it shows in the quality of the overall work. Dr Bethoux currently serves as the Director of Rehabilitation Services at the Cleveland Clinic, Mellen Center for Multiple Sclerosis Treatment and Research.

The first article is "Pathophysiology of Gait Disturbance in Neurologic Disorders and Clinical Presentations," authored by two distinguished faculty from the Gait and Motion Analysis Laboratory at the prestigious Moss Rehabilitation Center in Philadelphia, Drs Theera Vachranukunkiet and Alberto Esquenazi. Dr Esquenazi is the Chairman of the Department of Physical Medicine and Rehabilitation, in addition to being the Director of the Gait and Motion Analysis Laboratory at the prestigious Moss Rehabilitation Center in Philadelphia.

The second article, "Measuring Ambulation in Adults with Central Neurologic Disorders," is authored by Karen J. Nolan, PhD, Mathew Yarossi, MS, and Arvind Ramanujam, MS. Dr Nolan is a Research Scientist in the Human Performance and Movement Analysis Laboratory at Kessler Foundation Research Center. She has extensive experience in research involving lower extremity 3D movement analysis and pedobarography in patients with acquired brain injury. Her primary research interests involve using a technology-oriented approach to develop objective assessments and measure changes in functional mobility after orthotic and clinical intervention. Dr Nolan is the principal investigator on a multicenter clinical trial investigating neuroprosthetics for ambulation in stroke survivors.

Phys Med Rehabil Clin N Am 24 (2013) xi–xiii
http://dx.doi.org/10.1016/j.pmr.2012.12.002
1047-9651/13/$ – see front matter © 2013 Published by Elsevier Inc.

Following is an article on "Gait Analysis for Poststroke Rehabilitation: The Importance of Ground Reaction Forces and the Impact of Gait Speed," authored by our esteemed editor, Dr Bethoux, and his colleagues, Sylvie Nadeau and Martina Betschart.

"Rehabilitation of Ambulatory Limitations" appears next and is coauthored by Lara A. Pilutti and Audrey L. Hicks. Dr Hicks is also an internationally recognized researcher. Her work focuses on exercise rehabilitation in people with multiple sclerosis, spinal cord injuries, or advanced age, exploring the myriad benefits of increased physical fitness. Using techniques such as muscle biopsies, ultrasound imaging, EMG, and transcranial magnetic stimulation , her work has helped our understanding of the mechanisms underlying exercise-induced improvements in strength or function in these special populations.

Next is the article "Assistive Devices for Ambulation" by Joan E. Edelstein, MA, PT, FISPO, CPed. Professor Edelstein's day job is teaching students in the physical therapy doctoral program in this very area and she provides a remarkably thorough, user-friendly article.

"Technological Advances in Interventions to Enhance Poststroke Gait" is authored by Drs Lynne R. Sheffler and John Chae from the MetroHealth Medical Center. Dr Chae is known all over the world for his work on electrical stimulation in stroke patients. He was recently elected to the Institute of Medicine of the National Academies, a rare honor reserved for only a small percentage of esteemed academicians and researchers. Dr Sheffler, also faculty at Case Western Reserve University School of Medicine, and Dr Chae provide us with an up-to-date, comprehensive look at how far we have come in helping stroke survivors maintain walking.

Dr Robert W. Motl, an Associate Professor of Kinesiology at the University of Illinois at Urbana-Champaign, discusses "Ambulation and Multiple Sclerosis" in the next article. Touching on all aspects of a functional gait, he gives us useful tips that we can use to help our multiple sclerosis patients maintain walking. Dr Motl's research interests include pain, spasticity, neural structure and function, social-cognitive variables, disability, and quality of life.

The next article is "Measurement and Treatment of Imbalance and Fall Risk in Multiple Sclerosis Using the International Classification of Functioning, Disability, and Health Model" written by Michelle Cameron, MD, PT and Ylva Nilsagård, PT, PhD. Dr Cameron has looked at these areas as both an internationally recognized physical therapist, and then, following her return to medical school and subsequent postdoctoral training, a physician and neurologist. Ylva Nilsagård, PT, PhD, has studied using self-reported measures to help identify people with multiple sclerosis at increased risk for falls and other trauma. They provide a thorough overview of this area and show us how we can decrease the risk of falls in these patients.

Our issue concludes with articles focusing on ambulation in two different disorders: spinal cord injury and Parkinson disease. Drs Elizabeth C. Hardin, Rudi Kobetic, and Ronald J. Triolo coauthor the article, "Ambulation and Spinal Cord Injury." Dr Hardin brings her skills as a scientist at the Veteran's Medical Center in Cleveland, where she has been principal investigator on a grant project on neural prostheses and gait performance. Drs Kobetic and Triolo are also widely published in this area.

"Ambulation and Parkinson Disease" is authored by Drs Shinichi Amano, Ryan T. Roemmich, Jared W. Skinner, and Chris J. Hass, all esteemed researchers. The lead author, Dr Amano, has particular interests in the postural control of gain and balance in persons with Parkinson disease.

As always, I express my sincerest thanks and gratitude to all of the authors who put tremendous effort into making this a truly outstanding collection of up-to-date, cutting-edge articles that will help all of us provide the absolute best care to our patients with CNS neurodegenerative disorders. My congratulations also to our editor, Dr Francois Bethoux, for putting this together.

Gregory T. Carter, MD, MS
Muscular Dystrophy Association
Regional Neuromuscular Center
Providence Medical Group
Department of Clinical Neurosciences
Physical Medicine and Rehabilitation Division
410 Providence Lane, Building 2
Olympia, WA 98506, USA

E-mail address:
gtcarter@uw.edu

Preface

Ambulation in Adults with Central Neurologic Disorders

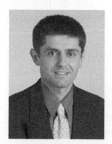

Francois Bethoux, MD,
Editor

"Walking is man's best medicine." This quote, attributed to Hippocrates, illustrates how long health care professionals have been interested in ambulation. The therapeutic effects of walking on the body and mind are mirrored by the ill effects of impaired ambulation and limited mobility in the environment. Many ailments can lead to walking limitations, and the effects of aging on walking have been well described. At the same time, walking performance has been identified as a marker or predictor of general health, to the point that the assessment of self-selected walking speed has been proposed as the "sixth vital sign" in elderly individuals.

Central neurologic disorders (including congenital disorders, diseases, and injuries) represent a particularly challenging cause of impaired ambulation: walking limitations are usually the result of multiple neurologic impairments, and the situation is often further complicated by comorbidities, as well as psychosocial and environmental factors, and sometimes the side effects of treatments. Too often, there is no cure for central neurologic disorders, and most of the chronic damage caused to the central nervous system cannot yet be repaired. Furthermore, some of these disorders are progressive, making even maintenance of functional performance a struggle.

However, advances in various fields present us with rapidly growing opportunities to fight the consequences of central neurologic disorders on ambulation. The International Classification of Functioning, Disability, and Health provides us with a conceptual framework to describe and assess these consequences beyond the traditional biomedical model. New exercise and rehabilitation techniques, medications, and devices are being developed. Assessment techniques give health care professionals a better understanding of the pathophysiology of gait disturbances and allow them to measure ambulation limitations, as well as the results of various interventions, from the gait laboratory to the environment, including self-report measures that directly capture the experience and concerns of individuals.

Phys Med Rehabil Clin N Am 24 (2013) xv–xvi
http://dx.doi.org/10.1016/j.pmr.2012.11.006
1047-9651/13/$ – see front matter © 2013 Published by Elsevier Inc.

pmr.theclinics.com

The goal of this issue is two-fold: to provide the base of knowledge needed to understand the latest developments related to the pathophysiology, assessment, and rehabilitation of ambulation limitations in central neurologic disorders, and to provide up-to-date information regarding the management of walking limitations in specific disorders, including stroke, multiple sclerosis, Parkinson disease, and spinal cord injury. We hope that these articles will provide readers with information that they can use in their own practice, will entice them to learn more on this very important topic, and will drive some to contribute to the body of knowledge through further research and publications.

Francois Bethoux, MD
Director, Rehabilitation Services
The Mellen Center for Multiple Sclerosis Treatment and Research
The Cleveland Clinic Foundation
9500 Euclid Avenue/Desk U10
Cleveland, OH 44195

E-mail address:
BETHOUF@ccf.org

Pathophysiology of Gait Disturbance in Neurologic Disorders and Clinical Presentations

Theera Vachranukunkiet, MD*, Alberto Esquenazi, MD

KEYWORDS

- Gait • Neurophysiology • Spastic gait • Ataxic gait • Parkinsonian gait

KEY POINTS

- This article reviews normal neural control of human ambulation.
- This article reviews basic kinematics and kinetics of normal human gait.
- This article describes pathophysiology and clinical presentation of spastic hemiparetic and paraparetic, ataxic, and Parkinsonian gait patterns.

NEURAL CONTROL OF NORMAL HUMAN AMBULATION

The neural control required to coordinate the complex motor output of normal human gait is still the topic of significant research. Much of the current understanding is based on animal studies, which have been extrapolated to humans. Animal studies have identified the existence of central pattern generators (CPGs) for ambulation, located in the spinal cord. These CPGs are neural networks that are capable of creating a motor pattern, independent of any sensory input.[1]

The CPG in human locomotion is able to incorporate afferent input from multiple sources to initiate and modify the basic motor pattern of gait and effectively coordinate muscle activation between the 2 lower limbs and between the upper and lower limbs. Voluntary changes in gait, such as change of speed/direction or avoiding an obstacle, seem to be modulated by supraspinal afferents. Reflexive changes in gait, such as stumble recovery, likely involve peripheral sensory afferents of cutaneous and muscle reflexes. There also seems to be differential control of flexor versus extensor muscle groups, with predominant central (supraspinal) control of the flexor muscle groups, and peripheral (proprioceptive) control of the extensor muscle groups.[2]

MossRehab Gait & Motion Analysis Laboratory, 60 Township Line Road, Elkins Park, PA 19027, USA
* Corresponding author.
E-mail address: theera_v@hotmail.com

Phys Med Rehabil Clin N Am 24 (2013) 233–246
http://dx.doi.org/10.1016/j.pmr.2012.11.010

Many supraspinal structures are involved in the control of ambulation, including the brainstem reticular formation; basal ganglia; motor, premotor, and supplementary motor area of the motor cortex; and cerebellum.[3,4] The midbrain locomotor region is involved in the initiation of locomotion based on its connections with limbic structures and the basal ganglia.[5] Basal ganglia interactions with the motor cortex via the cerebellum are involved in volitional motor control.[6] Basal ganglia thalamocortical interactions contribute to planning and execution of volitional movement.[7] Known pathways also exist between the basal ganglia and brainstem motor networks, but the precise role of the basal ganglia in controlling muscle tone and locomotion is not well understood.[8] From studies in Parkinson disease (PD), the basal ganglia seem to play a role in regulating step length and the timing of internal cues for each step.[9]

The cerebellum is involved in the coordination of limb movement and overall balance control. The medial cerebellar zone integrates spinal and vestibular inputs (ie, vestibulospinal and reticulospinal tracts), and helps to regulate extensor tone, maintain upright stance and dynamic balance control, and to modulate the rhythmic flexor and extensor muscle activity of locomotion. The intermediate cerebellar zone integrates spinal (dorsal spinocerebellar tract, ventral spinocerebellar tract) and cortical inputs, and helps direct limb placement and regulate agonist-antagonist muscle pairs, playing a key role in controlling the relative timing, amplitude, and trajectory of limb movements, particularly when precision is desired. The lateral cerebellum influences walking via cortical (motor, premotor, somatosensory) interactions and helps make adjustments to the normal locomotor pattern in novel or complex conditions or when strong visual guidance is required.[10]

The most significant sensory afferents for locomotion are from the visual, vestibular, and proprioceptive systems.[11] In addition to modulating the CPG, these afferents also interact with each other. For example, studies have shown that visual inputs decrease muscle spindle activity,[12] and that somatosensory loss can increase sensitivity of the vestibulospinal system.[13]

Proprioceptors located in tendons, muscles, ligaments, and joints relay information regarding limb position and kinesthesia. The dorsal column-medial lemniscus system relays sensory information (localized touch, pressure, vibration, and joint position sense) from the limbs to the sensory cortex. Proprioceptive information transmitted to the cortex assists with controlling volitional movements planned by the motor cortex. The dorsal spinocerebellar tracts relay information from muscle stretch and tension nerve fibers (ie, Golgi tendon organs, muscle spindles) to the cerebellum, and the ventral spinocerebellar tracts relay information from the spinal cord interneurons to the cerebellum. Proprioceptive information transmitted to the cerebellum assists with involuntary modulation of motor control.[14]

Load information carried by mechanical receptors in the sole of the feet and from proprioceptive inputs in the extensor muscles of the foot,[15] and afferents that signal hip-joint position,[16] play a role in leg muscle activation pattern and stance-swing phase transitions during ambulation. For example, excitation of muscle tendon organs in stance contribute to maintaining the stance phase while the limb is loaded, and may also help modulate that activity according to the load carried by the limb.[17]

NORMAL HUMAN AMBULATION

Simply stated, the goal of ambulation is to move the body mass from point A to B safely (ie, without falling). This section describes dynamic stability: maintaining upright posture and the body's center of mass within a moving base of support. When walking, there are periods of double support when both lower limbs are in contact with the ground, and periods of single support when only one limb is in contact with the ground. During single support, the body's mass moves from being relatively posterior to the supporting limb to anterior, and then alternates being supported by one limb and then the other.

Stance describes the phase in which the lower limb is in contact with the ground. The goals of the stance phase are to maintain stability while supporting body weight and to propel the body forward. Only after weight has been successfully transferred onto the stance limb can the swing phase begin on the contralateral side. Swing describes the phase in which the lower limb is in the air. The goals of the swing phase are to clear the limb over the ground while maintaining forward advancement of the center of mass, and to prepare the limb for the subsequent stance phase. At the basis of ambulation is this phasic cycling of stance and swing, alternating from one lower limb to the other. This basic pattern can be modified in either a proactive or a reflexive manner to meet a particular goal or accommodate differing environmental conditions.

The human gait cycle has been divided into different subphases (**Fig. 1**).

These subphases are useful when observing gait, and particularly when describing the relative timing of an observed deviation or problem. The motion of the key joints of the lower limbs during each of the subphases of gait has also been well described (**Fig. 2**). Understanding of normal kinematics is useful when describing not only the timing but also the nature of a gait deviation through indicating the problem joint and posture.

The coordinated patterns of muscle activation during gait are also well described. It is important to recognize that the recording of electromyogram (EMG) activity does not correlate with muscle strength or in some instances even movement, and thus these patterns provide only information about the timing of activation/termination of muscle activity. These activation patterns are phasic in nature, and the timing of activation/termination of activity occurs during well-defined periods of the gait cycle. Abnormalities of muscle activation can include absence of activity, abnormal onset of activation (early or delayed), abnormal duration of activation (abbreviated or prolonged), and presence of abnormal activation pattern (nonphasic pattern, clonic pattern). When both agonist and antagonist muscles are simultaneously activated, this is termed *cocontraction*. **Fig. 3** describes the activation pattern of key muscles during the gait cycle.

Understanding the functional significance of these muscle activation patterns during gait is one of the most difficult concepts to grasp, most likely because practitioners are anatomically trained to think almost exclusively of muscle activity in terms of concentric muscle contraction patterns in an open chain (eg, gastrocnemius causes ankle

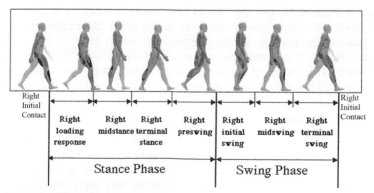

Fig. 1. Subphases of the gait cycle.

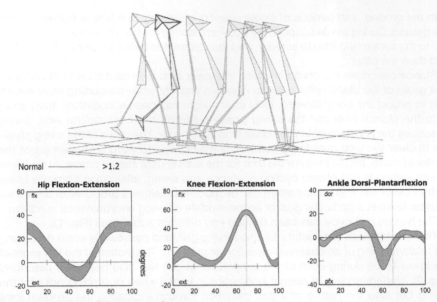

Fig. 2. Kinematics of the gait cycle.

plantarflexion, gluteus maximus causes hip extension). This knowledge can be applied in a fairly straightforward manner to the swing phase of the gait cycle. The foot is in the air, and therefore the observed joint movement is caused by active concentric muscle activation. However, the physics of inertia must also be considered. Although the hip flexion observed throughout swing phase is generated by concentric contraction of the hip flexors, the same is not true for the knee flexion observed during swing phase. In fact, the latter is largely passive, an inertial by-product of combined hip flexion and late-stance phase ankle plantarflexion.[18]

During the stance phase, the lower limb is in contact with the ground, forming a closed chain of activation. This mechanism allows muscles to influence joints that they do not cross, thereby increasing the complexity of the relationship between muscle activity and limb movement. For example, when the foot is fixed on the ground, the hip extensors are able to indirectly influence the knee joint, forcing it into extension by pulling the femur posteriorly. When the foot is fixed on the ground, this posterior motion of the femur forces the knee joint into extension passively. Similarly, in a closed chain, the ankle plantarflexors are able to force the knee into extension by pulling the tibia posteriorly. Although one of the roles of the ankle plantarflexors in gait is to generate push-off/propulsion via concentric contraction in late stance, the same muscles also contract isometrically and eccentrically earlier in the stance phase to control forward progression of the tibia, thereby playing a pivotal role in maintaining stance phase stability of the knee joint while minimizing quadriceps activity.[19]

CLINICAL PRESENTATIONS

Ambulation is the end result of a well-choreographed pattern of phasic muscle activation and deactivation, alternating between 2 lower limbs while transporting the superincumbent mass of the head, trunk, and arms. Given the multiple and complex neural pathways involved in producing ambulation, it is not surprising that disorders of the neurologic system can result in gait disturbance. In patients with neurologic disorders,

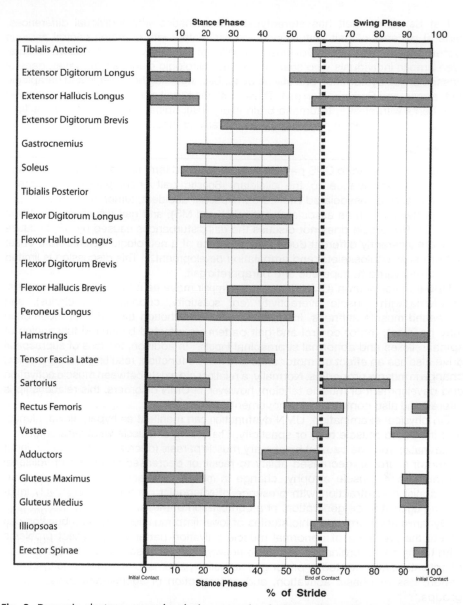

Fig. 3. Dynamic electromyography during normal velocity walking. Normal surface EMG activation pattern of key muscles during the gait cycle. (Normative *Data from* the MossRehab Gait & Motion Analysis Laboratory.)

gait disturbance is a manifestation of a primary problem that alters neural control of ambulation. Because normal pathways are disrupted, alternative means are required, and the net result is an abnormal pattern of locomotion. Importantly, the altered gait pattern that emerges is actually the body's attempt to achieve the goal of mobility via the use of remaining resources. In the absence of methods to correct the primary neurologic deficit, the goal of clinical gait evaluation and treatment is the optimization of available resources toward the goal of safe and efficient mobility.

Just as normal gait has stereotypic characteristics with individual differences, general patterns of gait disturbance are associated with common central nervous system (CNS) disorders. Obviously, significant variability of gait pattern occurs, even among individuals who share the same neurologic diagnosis; however, general classes of gait dysfunction can still be described, including hemiplegic and paraplegic gait, ataxic, and Parkinsonian gait. These patterns of gait dysfunction can be observed in patients with stroke, traumatic brain injury (TBI), spinal cord injury (SCI), multiple sclerosis (MS), cerebral palsy (CP), and PD, among others.

Spastic Gait

Spastic gait is linked to CNS pathology and is a broad term that is nondescriptive and of minimal significance to the clinician. Spastic gait encompasses hemiparetic patterns (such as associated with cerebrovascular accident, tumor, and TBI), paraparetic patterns (such as associated with SCI, and MS), and gait disorders in patients with CP. This article does not discuss the gait disturbances caused by CP, because they are inherently different due to the presence of a neurologic lesion before onset of normal musculoskeletal and ambulation development.[20] This discussion is limited to adult-acquired hemiparetic and paraparetic gait.

Upper motor neuron (UMN) lesions can impair movement through muscle paresis, problems with muscle overactivity (eg, spasticity, cocontraction, clonus), and increased muscle stiffness. In UMN lesions, even though the CPG for locomotion may be intact, motor control and gait pattern are affected by altered functioning of spinal reflexes and abnormal supraspinal inputs.[3] In addition, the loss of supraspinal drive also has an effect on motor units and muscle function, resulting in a mechanical change in muscle properties. Normally, a relationship exists between muscle activation and development of muscle tension; however, in UMN disorders, this relationship is altered and also contributes to movement disorder.[21]

On physical examination, UMN dysfunction can manifest as hyperreflexia, clonus, and increased muscle tone or spasticity. The finding of muscle weakness on clinical examination may be caused by primary muscle paresis (decreased descending input to motor neurons), decreased ability to recruit or decreased firing rate of volitional motor units,[22] muscle atrophy, change in muscle contractile properties, agonist-antagonist cocontraction with presence of antagonist contraction negatively influencing agonist force generation, or a combination of these.

Dynamic electromyographic studies of lower limb muscles during ambulation can reveal the presence of abnormal muscle activation patterns that reflect problems with timing and coordination of muscle activity, such as absent or reduced amplitude of activation, abbreviated or prolonged activation patterns, premature or delayed activation, loss of phasic activation, and cocontraction of agonist-antagonist muscle groups.[23,24]

Hemiparetic Gait

Observation of hemiparetic gait pattern reveals an overall marked loss of symmetry with a tendency for increased stance time on the unaffected limb. The normal reciprocal arm motion of gait is absent or diminished on the affected side, and may be flaccid in the early stages of recovery, or positioned in adduction and flexion. The affected lower limb seems stiff-legged, showing an extensor synergy pattern with extension, adduction, internal rotation of the hip; extension of the knee; and plantarflexion/inversion of the foot/ankle. Because of this extended limb posture, individuals have difficulty achieving adequate limb clearance during the swing phase, and observed compensatory maneuvers include hip hiking, lateral trunk sway (away from the affected limb), circumduction, and, less commonly, contralateral vaulting. Initiation of the swing phase is delayed, prolonged, or effortful, and usually associated with stiff-knee posture and ankle equinus (**Fig. 4**).

Compared with hemiparesis in stroke, gait in TBI has not been as well studied. The potential zone of neurologic insult in TBI is not nearly as well circumscribed compared with a stroke, and therefore results in a wider range of potential neurologic deficits. In one study, patients with TBI were shown to walk slower than normal subjects but faster than patients who had a stroke. This finding was attributed to increased step length generation compared with patients who had a stroke, and decreased step length on the unaffected side when compared with normal subjects. In contrast to patients who had a stroke, stance time for the affected limb was not prolonged, even though an increase in stance time was still seen on the unaffected limb.[25] The remainder of this discussion on hemiparetic gait refers to the stroke literature.

Studies of temporal-spatial parameters of ambulation in patients with hemiparesis after stroke have shown asymmetry with decreased stance and increased swing time on the affected side, increased stance time on the unaffected side when compared with the affected side, decreased step length on the affected side, and increased double support time. Overall, this pattern allows preservation of stability because increased time in double support and increased time weight-bearing on the sound limb result in decreased time weight-bearing on the affected limb.[26–28]

Speed of ambulation is decreased in patients with hemiparesis after stroke,[29] as is fastest comfortable walking velocity (ie, limited ability to increase speed of ambulation).[30] Studies have shown that muscle weakness of the hip flexors, knee extensors, and ankle plantarflexors is a key factor contributing to decreased speed of stroke ambulation, and also limited capacity to increase speed.[31–33]

Hemiparetic gait pattern in stroke has been evaluated via kinematic gait studies.[28] During the stance phase on the affected side, ankle dorsiflexion posture was

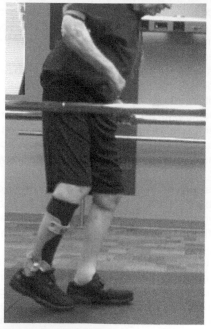

Fig. 4. Patient with right spastic hemiparesis.

decreased at initial contact and during stance and swing phases. Increased knee hyperextension in the stance phase was seen in most patients, although in some cases excessive knee flexion was observed. During the swing phase on the affected side, knee flexion was decreased, initiation of hip flexion was delayed, and compensation occurred via hip hiking (elevation of the hip) or limb circumduction. Kinetic studies have shown abnormally increased lateral plantar support, abnormal force transfer from hindfoot to forefoot with limited rollover, and reduced or absent push-off in terminal stance.[34]

Dynamic electromyographic studies of lower limb muscles during ambulation in patients who had a stroke reveal trends for prolonged total duration of tibialis anterior activity during the swing phase, overactivity in the gastrocnemius and soleus muscles during early stance, and coactivation of the quadriceps and hamstrings during stance.[23] Cocontraction of agonist-antagonist muscle groups has also been observed in patients who did not have a stroke (eg, patients with SCI or diabetic neuropathy, infants) and is thought to represent a compensatory strategy for stabilization of the limb.[23,35]

Paraparetic/Scissoring Gait

When bilateral upper motor neuron lesions occur, such as in patients with SCI or MS, the resultant bilateral lower limb involvement may or may not be symmetric. The typical spastic paraparetic gait is a bilateral stiff-legged gait pattern, often requiring the use of orthotic and/or assistive devices for ambulation. A scissoring pattern can be observed, in which increased activity of bilateral hip adductors causes the thighs to rub or the feet to cross each other during ambulation (**Fig. 5**). In the swing phase, excessive hip adduction can interfere with limb advancement and results in decreased width of base of support, with increased potential for impaired balance and falls. However, patients with hip flexor weakness may develop a compensatory strategy using the hip adductors as an alternative means to assist with limb advancement. This differentiation becomes particularly significant when considering treatment, because the elimination of increased hip adduction (eg, with botulinum toxin injections to decrease spasticity) may render patients nonambulatory if they have insufficient hip flexion for limb advancement.[36]

The degree of gait dysfunction in ambulatory patients with SCI depends on the level of injury and residual neurologic function, and factors such as muscle weakness, spasticity, and instability caused by impaired coordination and sensory deficits. Patients with thoracic level injuries were noted to have more spasticity and more abnormal gait parameters than those with lumbar cord injuries. Patients with thoracic cord lesions demonstrate reduced cadence, forward velocity, and knee angular velocity, whereas patients injured in the lumbar cord region have reduced stride length and ankle velocities.[37]

The degree of gait dysfunction in MS depends on the areas of injury and neurologic function. Patients may present with a combination of spastic and ataxic gait pattern, and studies have shown gait differences between patients with predominant pyramidal dysfunction and those with cerebellar dysfunction.[38] In patients with MS with early disease (patients with mild neurologic signs and no functional limitations), studies have confirmed the presence of gait and balance disturbance. Temporospatial abnormalities include reduced speed, increased double-support time, decreased stride length, decreased single-support time, and decreased swing time.[38–40] This pattern is observed in other diseases and likely reflects impaired balance and postural control. In early MS, kinematic changes in the ankle more than the knee joint have been observed, as has abnormally increased activation of the tibialis anterior and

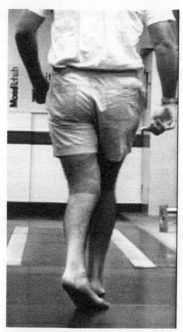

Fig. 5. Patient with adducted gait pattern.

gastrocnemius muscles during the swing phase. These altered muscle activation patterns were not attributable to slowed gait velocity, and likely reflect problems with impaired motor control.[41] Fatigue is also a significant issue during walking for patients with multiple sclerosis, and studies have shown decrease in both velocity and stride length over the course of a day.[42] The impact of other common neurologic impairments in MS, such as cognitive impairment and visual disturbance, has not been well studied.

Ataxic Gait

Ataxia comes from the Greek for "without order" and encompasses several different subtypes named for the neurologic system principally involved: cerebellar, sensory, vestibular, and mixed. Vestibular ataxia is associated with other signs and symptoms of vestibular dysfunction, such as nystagmus, vertigo, and nausea, and is characterized by a tendency to veer or deviate to one side during ambulation. Sensory ataxia is caused by proprioceptive sensory deficits, and is characterized by a staggering gait pattern exacerbated by ambulation on uneven surfaces in the dark or with eyes closed (positive Romberg). Secondary compensation in sensory ataxia can include stomping, slapping, or heavy heel strike at initial contact as a means to increase sensory feedback. An additional compensatory phenomenon is floor-seeking behavior in which the patient actively seeks visual input to compensate for proprioceptive deficits by looking to the feet/ground.

Cerebellar ataxia is caused by dysfunction of the cerebellum, which is involved in coordination of limb movement and dynamic balance control. Various anatomic zones of the cerebellum function in different ways: the medial zone regulates upright stance and dynamic balance, the intermediate zone modulates coordination and precision of limb movement, and the lateral zone influences locomotion when strong visual guidance is required or in complex situations. Thus, depending on the zones of cerebellar injury, the nature of gait disturbance may differ.

Cerebellar ataxic walking has been described as a "drunken" gait, which can be unstable, stumbling, veering, and irregular. Classically, an increased base of support is considered to be a key feature; however, temporospatial studies have provided inconsistent data regarding this particular gait parameter. Instead, current research has determined that the main feature of ataxic gait is increased intrasubject variability of performance.[43,44] More specifically, cerebellar disorders have increased timing variability that is not seen in other movement disorders with similar balance deficits and spatial variability.[45] For example, irregularity in the timing of peak flexion occurs at one joint with respect to other joints, or joint-joint decomposition in which multijoint movements are converted into a series of single-joint motions (**Fig. 6**).[10]

In addition, dynamic electromyographic studies have demonstrated abnormal cocontraction in the agonist-antagonist muscles of the distal leg during gait.[46] Cocontraction during limb movement reflects impairment of time-varying modulation, and results in problems performing precision movements. Performance of tandem gait, which requires precise foot placement, exacerbates gait disturbance in cerebellar ataxia and is a sensitive clinical test for cerebellar dysfunction.[47]

Parkinsonian Gait

PD is a specific disorder caused by deficiency of striatal dopamine, which results in impairment of basal ganglia function. The primary clinical deficit is hypokinesia, or slowness of movement, especially for volitional activity. Parkinsonian gait pattern is not specific to PD, and can also be observed in other processes that affect basal

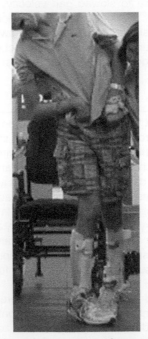

Fig. 6. Uncoordinated gait in a young subject after traumatic brain injury, requiring assistance for balance.

ganglia function and the frontal lobes. This pattern is sometimes also referred to as *hypokinetic-rigid gait pattern*.

The observed characteristics of Parkinsonian gait are a shuffling pattern with reduced step height, slow speed, and reduced reciprocal arm swing bilaterally. Delay occurs in initiation and termination of gait. Postural reactions are delayed in response to external challenge, with a potential increase in falls. Turns are difficult to perform and may be accomplished en bloc, via movement of the entire body. *Festination* refers to a gait pattern consisting of small rapid steps required to maintain the pedal base of support underneath the forward advancing body, and is observed in advanced disease.[48]

Monosynaptic and polysynaptic reflexes of distal leg extensors and the preprogrammed responses of flexor muscles are impaired in PD.[49] Polyelectromyographic studies show reduction in EMG activity in distal leg muscles compared with normal subjects.[46]

Temporospatial studies of ambulation in PD have shown nonspecific compensatory responses to gait dysfunction, including slow self-selected walking velocity, widened stance, decreased stride length, and an increased double-support period in relation to stride.[50–52] Kinematic studies have shown small angular displacement or decreased amplitude of leg movement that worsened with disease progression.[50] Quantitative studies have shown increased stride-to-stride variability of gait timing (ie, impaired ability to control timing from one stride to the next)[53] and problems with regulation of step length. Patients were shown to have normal or increased cadence for a given velocity, but impaired modulation of step length at different speeds.[54] Patients with PD have been shown to rely on visual input more than healthy controls, and the use of dopaminergic medications and visual and acoustic cues can partially reverse these deficits (**Fig. 7**).[55]

Apraxic Gait

Apraxic gait is defined as the loss of ability to use the legs for walking in the absence of sensory, motor, coordination, or other obvious impairment. Some controversy exists as to the use of the term *apraxia* in describing gait, because locomotion is not a skilled or learned motor act in strict definition. The terminology in the literature can also be confusing regarding these "higher order" gait disturbances, including Parkinsonism, marche a petit pas, Bruns ataxia, freezing of gait, gait ignition failure, and frontal gait.[56]

The overall presentation is that of a hypokinetic-rigid gait pattern, and people may have a general slowing of movements or may complain that their feet feel are "stuck to the ground." This phenomenon has also been termed *magnetic gait* because of the appearance of the feet being glued to the floor. Patients may also raise the leg in place without advancing the limb.

Apraxic gait is seen in patients with extensive cerebral damage, especially affecting the frontal lobes. An example is normal pressure hydrocephalus (NPH) in which problems with walking, progressive mental impairment and dementia, and impaired bladder control leading to urinary frequency and/or incontinence are clinical indicators. In September 2005 an international team of scientists developed clinical guidelines to help physicians diagnose NPH.[57] Similar symptoms are seen in other disorders, such as Alzheimer disease, PD, and Creutzfeldt-Jakob disease.

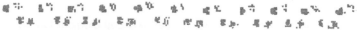

Fig. 7. GaitMat data set showing foot-fall pattern of patient with Parkinsonian gait pattern.

SUMMARY

Neurologic control of human ambulation is complex and incompletely understood. Given the complex interactions required to achieve normal gait, it is not surprising that ambulation dysfunction is a common presentation of neurologic disorder, and this article reviews several common clinical presentations of gait dysfunction in CNS disorders. In addition to close observation of gait patterns, instrumented gait analysis, including kinematic, kinetic, and dynamic electromyographic data, are helpful from research and clinical perspectives. Future studies are crucial for improving understanding of neural control of ambulation, and for the planning and impact of clinical interventions to improve ambulation.

REFERENCES

1. Grillner S. Neurobiological bases on rhythmic motor acts in vertebrates. Science 1985;228:143–9.
2. Dietz V. Proprioception and locomotor disorders. Nat Rev Neurosci 2002;3(10): 781–90.
3. Dietz V. Neurophysiology of gait disorders: present and future applications. Electroencephalogr Clin Neurophysiol 1997;103:333–55.
4. Duysens J, Van De Crommert HW. Neural control of locomotion; part 1: the central pattern generator from cats to humans. Gait Posture 1998;7:131–41.
5. Armstrong DM. Supraspinal contribution to the initiation and control of locomotion in the cat. Prog Neurobiol 1986;26:273–361.
6. Middleton FA, Strick PL. Basal ganglia and cerebellar loops: motor and cognitive circuits. Brain Res Brain Res Rev 2000;31:236–50.
7. Alexander GE, Crutcher MD. Functional architecture of basal ganglia circuits: neural substrates of parallel processing. Trends Neurosci 1990;13:267–71.
8. Takakusaki K, Saitoh K, Harada H, et al. Role of basal ganglia–brainstem pathways in the control of motor behaviors. Neurosci Res 2004;50:137–51.
9. Iansek R, Huxham F, McGinley J. The sequence effect and gait festination in Parkinson's disease: contributors to freezing of gait? Mov Disord 2006;21(9): 1419–24.
10. Morton SM, Bastian AJ. Mechanisms of cerebellar gait ataxia. Cerebellum 2007; 6:79–86.
11. Dietz V, Baaken B, Colombo G. Proprioceptive input overrides vestibulo-spinal drive during human locomotion. Neuroreport 2001;12:2743–6.
12. Jones KE, Wessberg J, Vallbo A. Proprioceptive feedback is reduced during adaptation to a visuomotor transformation: preliminary findings. Neuroreport 2001;12:4029–33.
13. Horak FB, Hlavacka F. Somatosensory loss increases vestibulospinal sensitivity. J Neurophysiol 2001;86:575–85.
14. Schneider RJ, Kulics AT, Ducker TB. Proprioceptive pathways of the spinal cord. J Neurol Neurosurg Psychiatry 1977;40(5):417–33.
15. Dietz V, Duysens J. Significance of load receptor input during locomotion: a review. Gait Posture 2000;11:102–10.
16. Pang MY, Yang JF. The initiation of the swing phase in human infant stepping: importance of hip position and leg loading. J Physiol (Lond) 2000;528:389–404.
17. Pearson KG. Proprioceptive regulation of locomotion. Curr Opin Neurobiol 1995; 5:786–91.
18. Perry J, Burnfield J. Gait analysis: normal and pathological function. Thorofare (NJ): Slack Publishing; 2010.

19. Kepple TM, Lohmann Siegel K, Stanhope SJ. Relative contributions of the lower extremity joint moments to forward progression and support during gait. Gait Posture 1997;6:1–8.
20. Dietz V, Berger W. Cerebral palsy and muscle transformation. Dev Med Clin Neurol 1995;37:180–4.
21. O'Dwyer NJ, Ada L, Nielson PD. Spasticity and muscle contracture following stroke. Brain 1996;119:1737–49.
22. Frontera WR, Grimby L, Larsson L. Firing rate of the lower motoneuron and contractile properties of its muscle fibers after upper motoneuron lesion in man. Muscle Nerve 1997;20:938–47.
23. Den Otter AR, Geurts AC, Mulder T, et al. Abnormalities in the temporal patterning of lower extremity muscle activity in hemiparetic gait. Gait Posture 2007;25: 342–52.
24. Lamontagne A, Malouin F, Richards CL, et al. Mechanisms of disturbed motor control in ankle weakness during gait after stroke. Gait Posture 2002;15: 244–55.
25. Ochi F, Esquenazi A, Hirai B, et al. Temporal-spatial feature of gait after traumatic brain injury. J Head Trauma Rehabil 1999;14:105–15.
26. Brandstater ME, Debruin H, Gowland C, et al. Hemiplegic gait: analysis of temporal variables. Arch Phys Med Rehabil 1983;64:583–7.
27. Wall JC, Turbull GL. Gait asymmetries in residual hemiplegia. Arch Phys Med Rehabil 1986;67:550–3.
28. Olney SJ, Richards C. Hemiparetic gait following stroke. Part I: characteristics. Gait Posture 1996;4:136–48.
29. Hsu AL, Tang PF, Jan MH. Analysis of impairments influencing gait velocity and asymmetry of hemiplegic patients after mild to moderate stroke. Arch Phys Med Rehabil 2003;84:1185–93.
30. Beaman CB, Peterson CL, Neptune RR, et al. Differences in self-selected and fastest-comfortable walking in post-stroke hemiparetic persons. Gait Posture 2010;31:311–6.
31. Bohannon RW. Selected determinants of ambulatory capacity inpatients with hemiplegia. Clin Rehabil 1989;3:47–53.
32. Nadeau S, Arsenault AB, Gravel D, et al. Analysis of the clinical factors determining natural and maximal gait speeds in adults with a stroke. Am J Phys Med Rehabil 1999;78:123–30.
33. Jonkers I, Delp S, Patten C. Capacity to increase walking speed is limited by impaired hip and ankle power generation in lower functioning persons post-stroke. Gait Posture 2009;29(1):129–37.
34. Mayer M. Clinical neurokinesiology of spastic gait. Bratisl Lek Listy 2002;103(1): 3–11.
35. Lamontagne A, Richards CL, Malouin F. Coactivation during gait as an adaptive behavior after stroke. J Electromyogr Kinesiol 2000;10:407–15.
36. Esquenazi A. Evaluation and management of spastic gait in patients with traumatic brain injury. J Head Trauma Rehabil 2004;19(2):109–18.
37. Krawetz P, Nance P. Gait analysis of spinal cord injured subjects: effects of injury level and spasticity. Arch Phys Med Rehabil 1996;77:635–8.
38. Givon U, Zeilig G, Achiron A. Gait analysis in multiple sclerosis: characterization of temporal–spatial parameters using GAITRite functional ambulation system. Gait Posture 2009;29:138–42.
39. Martin CL, Phillips BA, Kilpatrick TJ, et al. Gait and balance impairment in early multiple sclerosis in the absence of clinical disability. Mult Scler 2006;12:620–8.

40. Benedetti MG, Piperno R, Simoncini L, et al. Gait abnormalities in minimally impaired multiple sclerosis patients. Mult Scler 1999;5:363–8.
41. Kelleher KJ, Spence W, Solomonidis S, et al. The characterisation of gait patterns of people with multiple sclerosis. Disabil Rehabil 2010;32(15):1242–50.
42. Morris ME, Cantwell C, Dodd K. Changes in gait and fatigue from morning to afternoon in people with multiple sclerosis. J Neurol Neurosurg Psychiatry 2002;72:361–5.
43. Morton SM, Bastian AJ. Cerebellar control of balance and locomotion. Neuroscientist 2004;10:247–59.
44. Palliyath S, Hallett M, Thomas SL, et al. Gait in patients with cerebellar ataxia. Mov Disord 1998;13:958–64.
45. Ilg W, Golla H, Their P, et al. Specific influences of cerebellar dysfunctions on gait. Brain 2007;130:786–98.
46. Mitomaa H, Hayashib R, Yanagisawab N, et al. Characteristics of parkinsonian and ataxic gaits: a study using surface electromyograms, angular displacements and floor reaction forces. J Neurol Sci 2000;174:22–39.
47. Stolze H, Klebe S, Petersen G, et al. Typical features of cerebellar ataxic gait. J Neurol Neurosurg Psychiatry 2002;73:310–2.
48. Snijders AH, van de Warrenburg BP, Giladi N, et al. Neurological gait disorders in elderly people: clinical approach and classification. Lancet Neurol 2007;6:63–74.
49. Dietz V, Berger W, Horstmann GA. Posture in Parkinson's disease: impairment of reflexes and programming. Ann Neurol 1988;24:660–9.
50. Knutsson E. An analysis of parkinsonian gait. Brain 1972;95:475–86.
51. Blin O, Ferrandez AM, Serratrice G. Quantitative analysis of gait in Parkinson patients: increased variability of stride length. J Neurol Sci 1990;98:91–7.
52. Ebersbach G, Sojer M, Valldeoriola F, et al. Comparative analysis of gait in Parkinson's disease, cerebellar ataxia and subcortical arteriosclerotic encephalopathy. Brain 1999;122:1349–55.
53. Hausdorff JM, Cudkowicz ME, Firtion R, et al. Gait variability and basal ganglia disorders: stride-to-stride variations of gait cycle timing in Parkinson's disease and Huntington's disease. Mov Disord 1998;13(3):428–37.
54. Morris ME, Iansek R, Matya TA, et al. The pathogenesis of gait hypokinesia in Parkinson's disease. Brain 1994;117:1169–81.
55. Dietz V, Zijlstra W, Prokop T, et al. Leg muscle activation during gait in Parkinson's disease: adaptation and interlimb coordination. Electroencephalogr Clin Neurophysiol 1995;97:408–15.
56. Zadikoff C, Lang AE. Apraxia in movement disorders. Brain 2005;128:1480–97.
57. Relkin N, Marmarou A, Klinge P, et al. Diagnosing idiopathic normal-pressure hydrocephalus. J Neurosurg 2005;57(3):S4–16.

Measuring Ambulation in Adults with Central Neurologic Disorders

Karen J. Nolan, PhD[a,b,*], Mathew Yarossi, MS[a,c], Arvind Ramanujam, MS[a]

KEYWORDS

- Ambulation • Rehabilitation • Measurement • Gait analysis • Walking speed
- Central neurologic disorder

KEY POINTS

- Examine strategies for appropriate measurements of ambulation in individuals with central neurologic disorder within three distinct environments: 1) clinical; 2) laboratory; and 3) community.
- Discuss common challenges and solutions for clinicians and researchers when selecting appropriate outcomes for measuring ambulation.
- Description of technology-driven assessment tools for measuring ambulation to obtain objective, quantifiable outcomes.
- Explore techniques and research related to measurement of quantitative and qualitative ambulation in the community for persons with central neurologic disorder.

INTRODUCTION

Throughout rehabilitation medicine, there is an emphasis on the ability to ambulate as a functional outcome and as an overall indicator of quality of life. When ambulation is affected by central neurologic disorders (CND), it is typically as a result of a combination of impairments and the compensatory strategies used to accommodate these impairments. Pathologic ambulation can result from impairments within a single

Disclaimers: None.
Grant Support: Supported by Kessler Foundation.
Declaration of Interest: The authors report no conflicts of interest. The authors alone are responsible for the content and writing of the paper.
[a] Human Performance and Engineering Laboratory, Kessler Foundation Research Center, 1199 Pleasant Valley Way, West Orange, NJ 07052, USA; [b] Department of Physical Medicine and Rehabilitation, University of Medicine and Dentistry of New Jersey - New Jersey Medical School, Newark, NJ 07103, USA; [c] Department of Rehabilitation & Movement Sciences, Graduate School of Biomedical Sciences, University of Medicine and Dentistry of New Jersey - New Jersey Medical School, Newark, NJ 07101, USA
* Corresponding author. Human Performance and Engineering Laboratory, Kessler Foundation Research Center, 1199 Pleasant Valley Way, West Orange, NJ 07052.
E-mail address: knolan@kesslerfoundation.org

Phys Med Rehabil Clin N Am 24 (2013) 247–263
http://dx.doi.org/10.1016/j.pmr.2012.12.001
1047-9651/13/$ – see front matter © 2013 Elsevier Inc. All rights reserved.

pmr.theclinics.com

system or within a combination of systems, such as musculoskeletal, neuromuscular, sensory/perceptual, and cognitive/behavioral.[1]

Functional ambulation is the extent to which an individual is capable and willing to move around in their environment.[2] Measuring ambulation is a complex task involving clinical expertise, laboratory technology, and the ability to translate information to a community setting.

Measuring ambulation can be challenging, because walking occurs in multiple environments and must be assessed at multiple time points to indicate improvement or decline. There is an added complexity, because, in a traditional clinical environment, a single numerical value or scale score is preferred to summarize a series of complex movements,[3] whereas in a laboratory environment, researchers typically prefer quantifiable continuous data, which allow for complex analysis of multiple outcome variables. Measuring ambulation in a community also presents unique challenges and often requires a combination of strategies to obtain valid outcomes.[4] This review examines strategies for appropriate measurements of ambulation in individuals with CND within 3 distinct environments: (1) clinical, (2) laboratory, and (3) community. The purpose of this article is not to provide an exhaustive list of the measures that can be used to assess ambulation but rather to describe the most frequently used measures and to discuss common challenges faced by clinicians and researchers in establishing an accurate picture of an individual's ability to ambulate.

MEASURING AMBULATION IN THE CLINICAL ENVIRONMENT

In a clinical environment, it is important to select measures that can evaluate changes in impairment, function, and performance.[3] Test selection is often dependent on nonclinical criteria such as cost, time to administer, and available equipment.[5] It is also important for the patient to understand the test instructions, because unfamiliarity with the test can alter performance and outcomes.[5] Some examples of typical clinical assessments commonly used for measuring ambulation can be found in **Table 1**.

The Functional Independence Measure (FIM) was designed to measure burden of care in multiple rehabilitation populations.[3] The scores are based on clinical observation of 18 items of activities of daily living (ADLs) (13 motor and 5 cognition items).[6] Although there are motor items associated with this measure (including 1 item labeled locomotion and 1 labeled stairs), the overall FIM score is often not sensitive enough to reflect improvements in ambulation (particularly in situations in which walking performance has improved without a change in the level of assistance needed). Previous research also revealed a ceiling effect, and the FIM shows poor sensitivity to change in individuals with better walking abilities.[13] The FIM is typically used to determine independence at admission and discharge from inpatient rehabilitation. Another example of a frequently used clinical measure of motor deficits is the Fugl-Meyer Motor Assessment, which has previously been shown to correlate with length of stay in inpatient rehabilitation, and has been found to be predictive of discharge FIM scores and performance in ADLs. The disadvantage of this measure is that it assesses only gross limb movement and not fine or complex movements or coordination. Both the FIM and Fugl-Meyer Motor Assessment as a whole do provide reliable information about the results of rehabilitation, but it is difficult to specifically determine if, and how much, ambulation has improved using either of these assessment tools.

The Ambulation Index (AI) is an ordinal rating scale designed to assess independent mobility by evaluating the time and degree of assistance required to walk 7.62 m (25 ft), as well as the ability to transfer.[8] Previous research has found the AI to be useful as a grouping variable when measuring ambulation in individuals with stroke.[14] The

Table 1
Outcomes for measuring ambulation in a clinical environment

Name of Scale	Description	Measurement
Functional Independence Measure[6]	A 7-level ordinal scale that describes stages of complete dependence to complete independence in performance of basic activities of daily living	Ordinal scores based on clinical observation
Fugl-Meyer Motor Assessment[7]	Evaluates movement, reflexes, coordination, and speed, derived from the Brunnstrom stages of poststroke recovery. Frequently used to measure motor deficits	Ordinal scores are based on clinical observation and observed movements
Ambulation Index[8]	An ordinal rating scale designed to assess independent mobility by evaluating the time and degree of assistance required to walk 7.62 m (25 ft). The scale ranges from 0 (asymptomatic and fully active) to 9 (restricted to wheelchair; unable to transfer independently)	Ordinal scores are based on clinical observation, including observed performance, and timed walking speed
Emory Function Ambulation Profile, Modified Emory Functional Ambulation Profile [9,10]	The time (s) to ambulate through 5 common environmental terrains with or without an assistive device or manual assistance	The sum of the time (s) required to complete the 5 tasks
Walking Tests (2-minute, 6-minute, 10-minute, and 12-minute)[3]	Distance walked in meters in a given time is measured to indicate performance	Distance walked (m)
Dynamic Gait Index[11]	A tool to assess gait, balance, and fall risk. Eight abilities are graded on a 4-point scale (0–3) from normal performance to severely impaired. The rating is based on the individual's ability to maintain a healthy gait pattern and pace, without deviating or stumbling	Ordinal scores are based on clinical observation and observed performance
Timed Up and Go[12]	The time (s) required to rise from an arm chair, walk 3 m, turn, walk back, and sit down again	A categorical scale based on the time (s) required to accomplish the described task
10-m Walk Test, Timed 7.62 m (25-ft) Walk Test[3]	A measure of ambulation capacity including the time (s) to walk 10 m or 7.62 m (25 ft) at maximum but safe gait speed	Time and distance to calculate maximum gait speed (m/s)
Gait Speed[3]	The rate (s) a given distance (m) is covered to determine self-selected or fastest gait speed	Time and distance to calculate speed (m/s)

Adapted from Finch E, Brooks D, Stratford PW, et al. Physical rehabilitation outcome measures. 2nd edition. Ontorio (Canada): Lippincott Williams & Wilkins; 2002.

measure is useful in rehabilitation medicine, but it is not sensitive enough to measure small changes in ambulation. Overall, the FIM, Fugl-Meyer, and AI measure impairment and function but have limited usefulness in describing and evaluating ambulation.

When measuring ambulation in a clinical environment, it is important to consider that individuals with CND may have difficulty adapting to the demands of walking in the community, such as rising from a chair, stepping over an obstacle, ascending stairs, and navigating various terrains.[9] The challenge is to select tasks and terrains that mimic community ambulation that are easy to administer and provide relevant clinical information. The Emory Functional Ambulation Profile (EFAP) and the modified EFAP (mEFAP) were designed to provide quantitative information about ambulation by measuring the time to walk over a standardized array of community obstacles and surfaces, accounting for the use of assistive devices.[9,10] The EFAP and mEFAP are reliable and valid clinical tests of ambulation that are sensitive to changes in ambulation speed.[9,10] Research in individuals with stroke found that the mEFAP is sensitive to changes in gait function during inpatient rehabilitation and therefore could be used to supplement traditional subjective measures of clinical ambulation.[15]

Walking tests measure the distance walked in a given amount of time to indicate walking performance. These tests are generally 2, 6, 10, or 12 minutes in duration and are widely used in clinical and research applications for individuals with CND.[3] These measures are more quantitative and provide information directly related to ambulation, including walking endurance. Previous research in this area suggests that individuals must negotiate a distance of between 332 and 360 m to access goods and services in the community.[16,17] Walking distance is therefore a key indicator of ambulation.[18]

For individuals with CND, it is important to have clinical assessments that identify individuals who are at risk for falling and may benefit from interventions designed to improve balance.[19] The Dynamic Gait Index (DGI) was developed as a clinical tool to assess an individual's ability to modify gait in response to changing task demands.[11] The limitation of the DGI is that scores are reduced for those individuals using an assistive device, regardless of performance.[20] The DGI has been applied to individuals with CND as a reliable measure of dynamic balance and potential fall risk.[20,21] The Timed Up and Go (TUG) is a screening test of balance that is commonly used to evaluate functional mobility.[19] The time to complete the test is strongly correlated to the level of functional mobility. Adults who complete the TUG in less than 20 seconds are considered to be independent in transfer tasks associated with ADLs and can maintain walking speeds sufficient for community ambulation.[12,22]

In individuals with CND, alterations in gait mechanics, strength, and balance have a direct effect on gait speed.[5] The 10-m walk test and timed 7.62 m (25-ft) walk are measures of ambulation capacity in which gait speed is the primary outcome variable. These tests have been widely used in populations with CND and are easy to administer in a clinical environment.[3] When measuring ambulation, it is important for clinicians to select measures capable of detecting changes that reflect real life function.[23] Gait speed is an important and reliable measure of ambulation for individuals, because safe navigation of community crosswalks mandates that an individual be able to complete a prescribed distance in a defined time period.[16,23] Previous research in stroke found that when an ankle foot orthotic was worn on the paretic limb, individuals gained the ability to modulate gait speed. The orthotic intervention provided individuals with stroke with the functional ability to increase speed in the community, which is essential for negotiating obstacles and safely crossing community streets.[14,16] Gait speed is used in clinical and research applications as the hallmark of recovery, it is simple to implement, and it has robust psychometric properties.[24] Several studies have provided evidence to support the predictive validity of gait speed, and it has been shown to be positively correlated with level of disability, function, and quality of life in individuals with stroke.[25–27] However, what represents a clinically meaningful change in gait speed has not been defined in all patient populations.

MEASURING AMBULATION IN A LABORATORY ENVIRONMENT

In a laboratory, ambulation is measured using traditional clinical assessments in conjunction with technology-driven mobility assessment tools, to create quantifiable outcomes that can be used to describe mechanisms that may lead to improved ambulation. For example, increased gait speed may indicate improved ambulation, but does not necessarily indicate improved gait mechanisms or functional recovery. The goals of laboratory-based outcomes for measuring ambulation are to enhance traditional clinical measures, or to become fully integrated into routine clinical care to help direct treatment options and accurately measure changes in ambulation throughout the rehabilitation process.

History and Evolution of Measuring Ambulation

Gait is the way ambulation is achieved using human limbs, and gait analysis is the systematic evaluation of a person's walking pattern.[28] The origins of the science of gait analysis began in the seventeenth century in Europe, when scientists and researchers provided a solid scientific foundation of our current knowledge and the understanding of human ambulation.[29] Research in the twentieth century benefited from technological advancements, including the development of three-dimensional (3D) force plates, and kinesiological electromyography (KEMG), which moved the measurement precision of gait analysis significantly forward.[29] A summary of the evolution of these early techniques into the systems used today is described in **Table 2**.[29–31]

Although the early principles of gait analysis are recognized as the foundation of measuring ambulation, the methods used were too labor-intensive for practical application in a clinical setting.[29] Technology-driven systems for measuring ambulation continue to evolve in the laboratory, with the goal of translating these outcome measures into the clinical and community setting.

Techniques for Measuring Ambulation in a Research Laboratory

Gait analysis is a widely used measurement technique to assess, plan, and treat individuals with conditions affecting their ability to walk. Gait analysis emerges from the combined interaction of the human eye (image capture) and the human brain (image processing) used for recognition and identification of changes in ambulation.[32] A complete gait analysis can be achieved using visual observation to interpret human locomotion. Therapists frequently use observational gait analysis to evaluate patient ambulation, because instrumented measurement systems are not feasible during time-limited clinical visits. Observational gait analysis typically reveals compensations or impairments from underlying diseases but it is limited by the experience of the observer. Instrumented gait analysis is a more technical method that involves collection of quantifiable information through the use of cameras, force plates, electromyography (EMG), pressure sensors, and computer analysis to objectively measure an individual's walking pattern.[32] Quantitative state-of-the-art methods of analysis and equipment offer greater precision, specificity, and sensitivity to change. It is within the laboratory environment that the comparison of observational versus instrumented gait analysis must continue to be explored to advance clinical outcomes.

Healthy walking is the standard against which disease is measured. The key gait parameters that the clinician needs to compare against disease are described in **Table 3**.[1]

Table 2
Techniques for gait analysis: evolution and history

KEMG	J.R. Close, 1959	Studied the phasic action of muscles using a 16-mm movie camera with a sound track and was able to record single-channel muscle action potentials on cine film
	R.W. Vreeland and D.H. Sutherland, 1961	Used a 16-mm movie camera mounted on a turntable above an oscilloscope with a 3-channel EMG
	J.V. Basmajian, 1962	Developed the technique of inserting 2 very fine electrodes (50-μm) through a single small needle (fine-wire EMG)
	J.U. Baumann, 1974	Obtained an 8-channel Honeywell tape recorder with 6 channels for KEMG transmitted through telemetry
	S.R. Simon, 1977	Electromyography permitted simultaneous recording from 12 channels transmitted through a cable from subject to computer
	Current	Various commercially available multichannel surface and fine-wire EMG systems, including telemetered and wireless EMG capability and integrated software for comprehensive outcome analysis. Capable of measurements inside (clinical or laboratory) and outside (community) in various environments
Kinematics	M.P. Murray, 1964	Attached reflective targets to anatomic landmarks of subjects walking in illumination of strobe light
	P.V. Karpovich and G.P. Karpovich, 1959	Electrogoniometry
	R. Linder, 1965	Vanguard motion analyzer: developed methods to measure yaw, pitch, and roll using mathematical formulae, 2 or more cameras and a two-dimensional coordinate system
	E.H. Furnee, 1967–1989	Primas system: TV/motion analysis systems with automated recording of reflective marker positions
	Current	Multiple commercially available real-time optical motion capture systems with: (1) infrared HD cameras; (2) markerless motion capture; (3) active light-emitting diode technology; (4) wired and wireless systems and integrated software for comprehensive outcome analysis. Capable of measurements inside (clinical or laboratory) and outside (community) in various environments
Kinetics	M. Carlet, 1872	Developed and used air reservoirs to measure force applied to the heel and forefoot
	E.J. Marey, 1894	Developed first true force plate, which measured vertical component of ground reaction using a pneumatic mechanism
	J. Amar, 1916	Produced the world's first 3-component (pneumatic) force plate, *Trottoire Dynamique*
	J. Hawthorn, 1971	Dynamic force plate (piezoelectric force transducers)
	Current	Several multichannel force (6° of freedom) and pressure measurements systems. Capable of measurement in various environments indoors, outdoors. and under water

Adapted from Sutherland, DH, 2001, 2002, 2005 Refs.[29–31]

Table 3 Outcomes for measuring ambulation in a laboratory environment		
Spatial-temporal characteristics[33]	Spatial	Step length, stride length, step width, velocity, cadence
	Temporal	IDS (initial double support time), SS (single support time), TDS (terminal double support time), swing time
	Symmetry	Temporal-spatial symmetry ratios between limbs
Joint kinematics[34–36]	Rotations	3D joint angular rotations
	Angular velocities	Rate of change of 3D joint angles
	Center of mass	Excursion of the 3D center of mass
Joint kinetics[37]	Forces	3D joint forces (effect of ground reaction forces on joint motions)
	Torques	3D joint torques (a combination of joint rotations and forces)
EMG[37]	Muscle firing	EMG analysis to assess muscle activation patterns (timing and amplitude) as it relates to joint kinematics
	Co-contraction	Simultaneous activation of agonist and antagonist muscles, if any
Pedobarography[27,38,39]	Plantar pressures	Measuring the magnitude and timing of pressure acting between the plantar surface of the foot and a supporting surface to quantify loading, weight transfer, and area during walking

Measuring Ambulation Using Temporal-Spatial Characteristics

Temporal

Temporal parameters are calculated using the timing characteristics within a gait cycle, where each gait cycle is further divided into individual gait phases to make comparisons across several cycles. The complete gait cycle includes initial double support (the time between foot contact and contralateral toe off), single support (the time between contralateral toe off and contralateral foot contact), terminal double support (the time between contralateral foot contact and ipsilateral toe off), and swing (the time between ipsilateral toe off and ipsilateral foot contact).[33]

Spatial

Spatial parameters are measured using the linear measurements (displacement of markers) during a gait cycle. They include step length (the forward linear distance between the heel markers from foot contact to subsequent contralateral foot contact), stride length (the forward linear distance between the heel markers from foot contact to ipsilateral foot contact), and step width (the linear medial-lateral distance between heel markers from foot contact to contralateral foot contact).[33]

Symmetry

Symmetry measures are used to compare characteristics between the limbs.[33] Temporal-spatial gait symmetry indices are calculated using mean swing (seconds) and stance times (seconds) on both limbs to calculate the following variables: overall temporal symmetry; temporal swing symmetry; temporal stance symmetry; temporal swing stance symmetry; and spatial step symmetry (the ratio of step lengths on both limbs in millimeters). A normative range for temporal-spatial symmetry is assumed to be 0.9 to 1.1.[33] This technique has been effectively used in stroke to assess the behavior of the paretic and nonparetic limbs during gait, where an overall temporal symmetry value greater than 1 indicates a preference to rely on the nonparetic limb during walking.[33,40]

Quantifying Ambulation with Kinematic and Kinetic Analysis

Kinematic

Kinematic data consist of temporal, linear, and angular variables. They quantify the features of gait describing the movements of the body segments and joint angles: temporal (timing), linear (displacement), and angular measurements. Temporal data describe the stride duration and the limb coordination patterns. Distance data, computed from the coordinates of the markers, describe the stride length, the distances between limb placements, and the flight paths of the body parts. Angular data describe the displacements, velocities, and accelerations of the body segments and joints. Kinematic output from the motor control system is useful for measuring the movement variance during walking and helps to classify gait diseases.[36,41] **Fig. 1** shows sagittal plane joint angles at the hip, knee, and ankle during healthy walking.[42]

Motion capture systems in a laboratory setting are routinely used to measure ambulation by evaluating changes in gait kinematics. Reflective markers are placed on selected anatomic landmarks and captured with the use of infrared cameras in a 3D space. Data reduction and kinematic modeling can then be performed to calculate linear and angular measurements. The data may then be displayed graphically for presentation and report generation.[1,43] Deviations or changes in kinematics can help to identify and measure gait deficits, thereby initiating clinical interventions for rehabilitation. In an individual with CND, gait analysis may show unilateral or bilateral circumduction, abnormal pelvic movements, and a lack of ankle dorsiflexion during

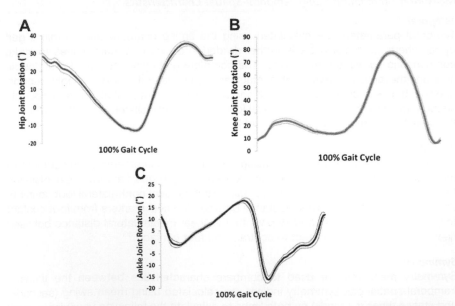

Fig. 1. Sagittal plane gait kinematics, during healthy adults walking: (*A*) hip, (*B*) knee, and (*C*) ankle. Each plot represents the mean ± standard deviation for 1 representative subject over 10 consecutive trials. (*Data from* Ramanujam A, Forrest GF, Sisto SA. Methological variability in evaluating gait dynamics: a comparative study. Gait and Clinical Movement Analysis Society 13th Annual Meeting. Richmond, Virginia, April 2-5, 2008. p. 278–9.)

swing (foot drop). After physical therapy or assistive device intervention, further kinematic testing can precisely measure changes in ambulation to direct future treatment strategies.[44]

Kinetic

Kinetic analysis measures forces, both external and internal to the body. Forces developed by muscles are transformed into rotations of the limb segments that produce movement. The ground reaction forces (GRF) during locomotion can be recorded using a force plate. Intrinsic joint forces and torques are then calculated from knowledge of the GRFs using inverse dynamic calculations. When an individual steps on the force plate, the force is detected by transducers or strain gauges and is converted to an electrical signal that is amplified and recorded. Variables measured by the force plate include the stance duration, the magnitude of the vertical, longitudinal (horizontal craniocaudal), and transverse (horizontal mediolateral) forces, the time when the peak forces occur, the impulses (area under the force time curves), and the point of application of the force (center of pressure). Displacement of the center of pressure has been evaluated for individuals with stroke and has been a robust measure to predict gait velocity, a reliable indicator of both pathologic gait and general functional status in rehabilitation.[45–47]

Normal forces plantar to the foot during walking can also be measured using pressure sensor technology, such as insole sensors or pressure mats. Measuring changes in loading during ambulation provides quantitative information that cannot be obtained without instrumentation. This technology has been used to evaluate weight transfer, an analytical method that quantifies linearity of loading and transfer of momentum during gait. These outcome variables have been used to evaluate orthotic intervention and are significant factors related to the improvement of ambulation.[39]

Use of EMG

EMG provides information on the state of activity of the motor neurons at rest, during reflex contraction, and during voluntary contraction. During ambulation, muscular contraction generates forces that stabilize and move the limbs. This process is preceded by electrical activation, which can be detected and recorded as the EMG. EMG signals are used in clinical and laboratory environments as a diagnostic tool to identify neuromuscular diseases and disorders of motor control. When measuring ambulation, the outcome variables obtained from EMG analysis provide quantifiable information about the coordination of complex muscle movements and can show mechanisms to compensate for muscle weakness.[48] Recent research investigating the use of a peroneal nerve stimulator in individuals with stroke found increased muscle activation during gait. Use of EMG provided information about therapeutic gains after intervention that extended beyond the ankle joint and the typically measured increase in dorsiflexion angle.[49]

Measuring Energy Consumption in a Research Laboratory

Individuals with CND who experience difficulty with ambulation typically also have an increased energy cost during walking. Decreased walking speed associated with CND contributes to reduced gait efficiency by preventing efficient energy transfer.[50] Previous research has suggested that faster walking speeds promote a more cost-effective gait pattern.[50,51] A straightforward method of evaluating the energy cost of walking is the physiologic cost index (PCI). The PCI measures the effort involved in walking as an increase in steady heart rate during movement (compared with a resting state) divided by the velocity of that movement.[52] Research has suggested a linear relationship between heart rate during sustained walking and maximum oxygen consumption.[53] PCI can provide quantitative information of energy cost to any mobility assessment by adding a device to measure heart rate and velocity.

Alternatively, Vo_2 peak can be used as an indirect measure of an individual's peak aerobic capacity. Aerobic capacity has been defined as the maximal amount of physiologic work an individual can perform, measured by oxygen consumption.[54] Measurements of walking economy can estimate the energy demands of an individual and characterize physiologic capacity for exercise.[55] In a laboratory environment, measurement of Vo_2 and walking economy can be obtained using precise instrumentation and a standard treadmill.[56]

MEASURING AMBULATION IN THE COMMUNITY

Reintegration into the community and maintenance of ADLs are the goal of rehabilitation programs for persons with CND. In a free-living population, technology-driven ambulation assessment measures often cannot be effectively used because of the constraints of the home/community environment. Measurement of community ambulation involves an individual's interaction within their environment and therefore must take into account the psychosocial aspects of that interaction as well as the physical impairment.[4,57] It is the patient's home environment that sets the context for evaluations of individual goals as they relate to quality of life. Complex measures that are both qualitative and quantitative are required, making measurement of ambulation in the community perhaps the most challenging environment in which to define meaningful outcomes for measuring ambulation.[58]

Additional levels of complexity in measuring community ambulation are found in the interaction with other impairments such as cognition that affect spatial recognition, memory, and attention.[59,60] In clinical and laboratory environments, there is diminished attention paid to cognitive impairments, to focus on the effects of physical impairments on ambulation. In the community, an individual must be able to ambulate in combination with cognitive tasks, therefore the cognitive and physical are interrelated when measuring community ambulation.[22,61,62] Although several clinical measures have been developed to simulate community ambulation activities, such as those requiring gait over uneven surfaces or dual task assessments requiring additional cognitive or attentional involvement during gait, the ability to measure the interaction with other impairments in real situations in the community are virtually nonexistent.

Previous research has concentrated on several areas related to measurement of mobility impairment in the community such as measurement of impairment, activity, participation, and quality of life.[4] The following section highlights several of the important techniques and findings related to measurement of ambulation in the community for persons with CND.

Qualitative Measurements of Ambulation

Most often, qualitative measurements of community ambulation are obtained through the use of self-report survey instruments that seek to categorize an individual's ability to ambulate in different situations. Measures of community ambulation and participation are often aimed at categorically identifying the ADLs that an individual is capable of performing, as well as the level of assistance needed, in terms of use of assistive devices and care from another person.

In the population with stroke, both Perry and colleagues[46] and Lord and colleagues[61] have conducted studies in which participants rated their ability to perform such tasks as getting to appointments or walking from their homes to the mailbox. Based on their ability to accomplish such tasks independently, participants were classified as noncommunity, limited community, or full community ambulators.

In a 2005 review, Lord and colleagues[61] described many of the classification schemes to assess community participation in stroke such as the Subjective Index of Physical and Social Outcome,[63] the Reintegration to Normal Living Index,[64] the Sickness Impact Profile,[65] the Frenchay Activities Index,[66] the Nottingham Extended Activities of Daily Living Index,[67] and the Stroke Impact Scale.[68] The Unified Parkinson's Disability Rating Scale is the gold standard instrument used to measure disease severity in Parkinson disease and includes questions about the ability to successfully ambulate in various community environments.[69] Although these scales have been validated for the classification of community ambulation ability, few could be considered measurement tools that can successfully assess the quantity or quality of ambulation in the community. The Spinal Cord Injury-Functional Index measurement system uses a 5-factor model, comprising basic mobility, ambulation, wheelchair mobility, self-care, and fine motor function, with the goal of comprehensively assessing physical function for individuals with spinal cord injury.[70]

Although many of these classification systems are specific to 1 population, the International Classification of Functioning (ICF) from the World Health Organization[71] has been used across many populations with CND. The ICF has multiple components that aim to assess the way an individual's disability affects all aspects of life. To assess the effect of limited community ambulation, as it relates to overall quality of life, the ICF uses 3 domains: (1) body functions and structures (impairment); (2) activity; and (3) participation.[72] Using this framework, deficits in the ability to ambulate in the community can be categorized as impairments of body functions and structures (such as weakness or pain), environmental factors (including accessibility of the home and available transportation), as well as personal factors (including motivation and support). Included in this assessment are questions about self-efficacy, which represents the individual's perception of their own ability. Often individuals avoid activities that they perceive are too difficult, and therefore it is important to understand the perception of disability when evaluating the effect of disability as a whole.[71] The goal of the ICF is to provide a framework that considers not only physical impairment but also social barriers to accurately classify community ambulation.[71,72]

Other broadly used scales across multiple populations are the Ambulatory Self-Confidence Questionnaire,[73] aimed at specifically examining self-efficacy, which has been used in patient populations with both Parkinson disease and multiple sclerosis. The Environmental Analysis of Mobility Questionnaire, developed in nonneurologically impaired geriatric populations, has also been validated to study community ambulation in persons with CND.[62,74]

Quantitative Measurements of Community Ambulation

Quantitative measurements of community ambulation provide more reliable outcomes, compared with qualitative measures, when used in various populations with CND. Many of the laboratory technologies described earlier cannot be used in the community. Often, assessments of community ambulation must depend on comparatively simple technologies that result in different outcomes/goals from those of laboratory and clinical assessments. Unlike in the laboratory, where greater specificity and detail are paramount, community-based technologies must be able to collect data for long periods and not impede ADLs.[75] However, the need to understand commonly used clinical and laboratory ambulation measures is essential to effectively adapt quantitative measures to evaluate community outcomes.

Common technologies used for quantitative assessment of community ambulation include pedometers, accelerometers, and GPS (Global Positioning System)-based devices.[58,75] The goal of these instruments is to provide long-term, remote, unobtrusive monitoring of ambulatory activity.[76,77] It is also important to provide data on a timescale that allows the observation of changes in activity patterns.[78]

Pedometer-based activity monitors report data as number of steps per unit time using sensors that measure a combination of acceleration, position, and time (**Fig. 2**). Outcome measures include daily step counts, measures of peak activity, stepping bout duration quantified by the amount of time spent continuously stepping, and the amount of time ambulating at predefined activity levels.[77] In a study of individuals with chronic hemiplegia secondary to stroke, Roos and colleagues[79] found that those with a self-reported status of "unlimited community ambulators" ambulated more in the community than "limited community ambulators." Ambulation by all participants was found to be in short bouts, and sustained ambulation was uncommon.[75,79] Using similar techniques in individuals with Parkinson disease to assess declines in community ambulation, Cavanaugh and colleagues[80] found that participants had significant declines in the amount and intensity of daily ambulatory activity, but not in its frequency and duration. This research indicates that it is not only important to assess the amount of ambulation in terms of step counts or distance traveled but also to track the variation in day-to-day ambulatory activity. **Fig. 2** shows a sample of data from an accelerometer-based activity monitor, representing steps taken per day for 1 individual with stroke and an analysis of community ambulation by intensity for 17 participants with foot drop secondary to stroke.[78]

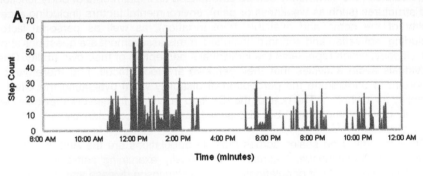

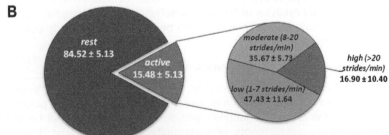

Fig. 2. Sample community ambulation data from an accelerometer-based activity monitor. (*A*) One representative day of total steps taken for 1 subject with stroke; (*B*) daily community ambulation data analyzed by intensity for 17 participants with foot drop secondary to stroke. (*Data from* Yarossi M, Franco B, Nolan KJ. StepWatch measures of community ambulation in individuals with hemiplegia following stroke. Archives of Physical Medicine and Rehabilitation–ACRM/ASNR Annual Conference 2011;92(10):1720.)

Reports of agreement between self-report and objective measures of community ambulation are mixed.[61,81] Average daily steps were measured for individuals with chronic incomplete spinal cord injury (n = 50), and a significant difference was found between self-reported community and noncommunity walkers.[81] In contrast, a study by Lord and colleagues[61] concluded that persons with stroke showed greater activity on self-report measures than what was measured objectively. Self-report measures inherently depend on an individual's perception of their own health and impairment and are often useful only in the context of the individual and are difficult to evaluate at the group level.

Understanding the strength of the relationship between commonly used clinical and laboratory measures and ambulatory activity in the community is essential for the use of clinical measurement to predict community outcomes. Research in chronic stroke reported on correlation and predictive ability of several clinical measures of ambulation including the Rivermead Mobility Index, Rivermead Motor Assessment, 6-minute walk test (6MWT), 10-m walk test (10MWT), and data collected from step activity monitors (SAM) worn in the community by participants with chronic stroke.[77] Only the 6MWT and the 10MWT were found to correlate with SAM data, and only the 6MWT was a significant predictor of step counts. In recent research in individuals with stroke, step activity was analyzed by intensity (see **Fig. 2**), and no significant relationships were found between clinical measurements of gait speed and endurance (timed 7.62-m [25-ft] walk and 6MWT), the number of steps taken per day, or the amount of the day spent active.[78,82] Clinical measures were correlated to measures of peak activity only during community ambulation, which indicated that individuals with hemiplegia who were able to sustain activity greater than 20 steps per minute walked more in the community.[78] Future work to better understand and measure community ambulation will have a valuable impact when evaluating individuals for treatment, which will provide more independence in performing ADLs.

SUMMARY

The goal of most rehabilitation programs is successful reintegration into the community. The ability to accurately measure ambulation, one of the most important metrics used to show transition into a community environment, is essential to measure treatment effectiveness and rehabilitation outcomes in populations with CND.

Measurements of ambulation in populations with CND should: (1) be predictive of disease state or progression; (2) be useful for evaluating recovery or intervention; (3) be diagnostic; (4) indicate the need for assistance in the community; (5) be able to provide information related to quality of life; and (6) use state-of-the-art technology. In addition, measurements of ambulation should be carefully examined for administration within a particular environment (clinical, laboratory, or community). Even the most robust measure of ambulation is affected by the environment in which it is implemented. Type of measurement or environment selected depends on the clinical or research question and the specificity of the hypothesis investigated.

REFERENCES

1. Perry J, Burnfield JM. Gait analysis: normal and pathological function. 2nd edition. Thorofare (NJ): Slack; 2010.
2. Coleman KL, Smith DG, Boone DA, et al. Step activity monitor: long-term, continuous recording of ambulatory function. J Rehabil Res Dev 1999;36(1):8–18.
3. Finch E, Brooks D, Stratford PW, et al. Physical rehabilitation outcome measures. 2nd edition. Ontario (Canada): Lippincott Williams & Wilkins; 2002.

4. Lord SE, Rochester L. Measurement of community ambulation after stroke: current status and future developments. Stroke 2005;36(7):1457–61.
5. Jackson AB, Carnel CT, Ditunno JF, et al. Outcome measures for gait and ambulation in the spinal cord injury population. J Spinal Cord Med 2008;31(5): 487–99.
6. Keith RA, Granger CV, Hamilton BB, et al. The functional independence measure: a new tool for rehabilitation. Adv Clin Rehabil 1987;1:6–18.
7. Fugl-Meyer AR, Jaasko L, Leyman I, et al. The post-stroke hemiplegic patient. 1. A method for evaluation of physical performance. Scand J Rehabil Med 1975; 7(1):13–31.
8. Hauser SL, Dawson DM, Lehrich JR, et al. Intensive immunosuppression in progressive multiple sclerosis. A randomized, three-arm study of high-dose intravenous cyclophosphamide, plasma exchange, and ACTH. N Engl J Med 1983; 308(4):173–80.
9. Wolf SL, Catlin PA, Gage K, et al. Establishing the reliability and validity of measurements of walking time using the Emory Functional Ambulation Profile. Phys Ther 1999;79(12):1122–33.
10. Baer HR, Wolf SL. Modified Emory Functional Ambulation Profile: an outcome measure for the rehabilitation of poststroke gait dysfunction. Stroke 2001;32(4): 973–9.
11. Shumway-Cook A, Woollacott M. Motor control: theory and applications. Baltimore (MD): Wilkins & Wilkins; 1995.
12. Podsiadlo D, Richardson S. The timed "Up & Go": a test of basic functional mobility for frail elderly persons. J Am Geriatr Soc 1991;39(2):142–8.
13. Cohen ME, Marino RJ. The tools of disability outcomes research functional status measures. Arch Phys Med Rehabil 2000;81(12 Suppl 2):S21–9.
14. Nolan KJ, Savalia KK, Lequerica AH, et al. Objective assessment of functional ambulation in adults with hemiplegia using ankle foot orthotics after stroke. PM R 2009;1(6):524–9.
15. Liaw LJ, Hsieh CL, Lo SK, et al. Psychometric properties of the modified Emory Functional Ambulation Profile in stroke patients. Clin Rehabil 2006;20(5):429–37.
16. Cohen JJ, Sveen JD, Walker JM, et al. Establishing a criteria for community ambulation. Top Geriatr Rehabil 1987;3(1):71–7.
17. Lerner-Frankiel MB, Vargas S, Brown M, et al. Functional community ambulation: what are your criteria? Clinical Management 1986;6(2):12–5.
18. Fulk GD, Echternach JL, Nof L, et al. Clinometric properties of the six-minute walk test in individuals undergoing rehabilitation poststroke. Physiother Theory Pract 2008;24(3):195–204.
19. Shumway-Cook A, Brauer S, Woollacott M. Predicting the probability for falls in community-dwelling older adults using the Timed Up & Go Test. Phys Ther 2000;80(9):896–903.
20. Jonsdottir J, Cattaneo D. Reliability and validity of the dynamic gait index in persons with chronic stroke. Arch Phys Med Rehabil 2007;88(11):1410–5.
21. McConvey J, Bennett SE. Reliability of the Dynamic Gait Index in individuals with multiple sclerosis. Arch Phys Med Rehabil 2005;86(1):130–3.
22. Smulders K, van Swigchem R, de Swart BJ, et al. Community-dwelling people with chronic stroke need disproportionate attention while walking and negotiating obstacles. Gait Posture 2012;36(1):127–32.
23. Fulk GD, Echternach JL. Test-retest reliability and minimal detectable change of gait speed in individuals undergoing rehabilitation after stroke. J Neurol Phys Ther 2008;32(1):8–13.

24. Tilson JK, Sullivan KJ, Cen SY, et al. Meaningful gait speed improvement during the first 60 days poststroke: minimal clinically important difference. Phys Ther 2010;90(2):196–208.
25. Goldie PA, Matyas TA, Evans OM, et al. Maximum voluntary weight-bearing by the affected and unaffected legs in standing following stroke. Clin Biomech (Bristol, Avon) 1996;11(6):333–42.
26. Schmid A, Duncan PW, Studenski S, et al. Improvements in speed-based gait classifications are meaningful. Stroke 2007;38(7):2096–100.
27. Nolan KJ, Yarossi M. Preservation of the first rocker is related to increases in gait speed in individuals with hemiplegia and AFO. Clin Biomech 2011;26(6):655–60.
28. Chambers HG, Sutherland DH. A practical guide to gait analysis. J Am Acad Orthop Surg 2002;10(3):222–31.
29. Sutherland DH. The evolution of clinical gait analysis. Part I: kinesiological EMG. Gait Posture 2001;14(1):61–70.
30. Sutherland DH. The evolution of clinical gait analysis. Part II: kinematics. Gait Posture 2002;16(2):159–79.
31. Sutherland DH. The evolution of clinical gait analysis. Part III: kinetics and energy assessment. Gait Posture 2005;21(4):447–61.
32. Whittle MW. Gait analysis an introduction. 4th edition. New York: Butterworth Heinemann; 2007.
33. Patterson KK, Parafianowicz I, Danells CJ, et al. Gait asymmetry in community-ambulating stroke survivors. Arch Phys Med Rehabil 2008;89(2):304–10.
34. Wu G, Siegler S, Allard P, et al. ISB recommendation on definitions of joint coordinate system of various joints for the reporting of human joint motion–part I: ankle, hip, and spine. International Society of Biomechanics. J Biomech 2002; 35(4):543–8.
35. Wu G, van der Helm FC, Veeger HE, et al. ISB recommendation on definitions of joint coordinate systems of various joints for the reporting of human joint motion–part II: shoulder, elbow, wrist and hand. J Biomech 2005;38(5):981–92.
36. Lee HJ, Chou LS. Detection of gait instability using the center of mass and center of pressure inclination angles. Arch Phys Med Rehabil 2006;87(4):569–75.
37. Winter DA. Biomechanics and motor control of human movement. 4th edition. Hoboken (NJ): John Wiley; 2009.
38. Soames RW. Foot pressure patterns during gait. J Biomed Eng 1985;7(2):120–6.
39. Nolan KJ, Yarossi M. Weight transfer analysis in adults with hemiplegia using ankle foot orthosis. Prosthet Orthot Int 2011;35(1):45–53.
40. Esquenazi A, Ofluoglu D, Hirai B, et al. The effect of an ankle-foot orthosis on temporal spatial parameters and asymmetry of gait in hemiparetic patients. PM R 2009;1(11):1014–8.
41. Burnfield JM, Powers CM. The role of center of mass kinematics in predicting peak utilized coefficient of friction during walking. J Forensic Sci 2007;52(6):1328–33.
42. Ramanujam A, Forrest GF, Sisto SA. Methodological variability in evaluating gait dynamics: a comparative study. Gait and Clinical Movement Analysis Society 13th Annual Meeting. Richmond, Virginia, April 2-5, 2008. p. 278–9.
43. Bensoussan L, Viton JM, Barotsis N, et al. Evaluation of patients with gait abnormalities in physical and rehabilitation medicine settings. J Rehabil Med 2008; 40(7):497–507.
44. Nolan KJ, Savalia KK, Yarossi M, et al. Evaluation of a dynamic ankle foot orthosis in hemiplegic gait: a case report. NeuroRehabilitation 2010;27(4):343–50.
45. Mizelle C, Rodgers M, Forrester L. Bilateral foot center of pressure measures predict hemiparetic gait velocity. Gait Posture 2006;24(3):356–63.

46. Perry J, Garrett M, Gronley JK, et al. Classification of walking handicap in the stroke population. Stroke 1995;26(6):982–9.
47. Nolan KJ, Yarossi M. Changes in COP displacement with the use of a foot drop stimulator in individuals with stroke 13th Emed Scientific Meeting (ESM). Aalborg, Denmark, August 1–4, 2012.
48. Brunner R, Romkes J. Abnormal EMG muscle activity during gait in patients without neurological disorders. Gait Posture 2008;27(3):399–407.
49. Yarossi M, Ramanujam A, Pilkar R, et al. Therapeutic gains after utilization of a foot drop stimulator in stroke extend beyond the ankle joint: a case report. Archives of Physical Medicine and Rehabilitation– ACRM/ASNR Annual Conference 2012;93(10):e19.
50. Lamontagne A, Stephenson JL, Fung J. Physiological evaluation of gait disturbances post stroke. Clin Neurophysiol 2007;118(4):717–29.
51. Hesse S, Werner C, Paul T, et al. Influence of walking speed on lower limb muscle activity and energy consumption during treadmill walking of hemiparetic patients. Arch Phys Med Rehabil 2001;82(11):1547–50.
52. MacGregor J. The evaluation of patient performance using long-term ambulatory monitoring technique in the domiciliary environment. Physiotherapy 1981;67(2):30–3.
53. Wieler M, Stein RB, Ladouceur M, et al. Multicenter evaluation of electrical stimulation systems for walking. Arch Phys Med Rehabil 1999;80(5):495–500.
54. Resnick B, Michael K, Shaughnessy M, et al. Inflated perceptions of physical activity after stroke: pairing self-report with physiologic measures. J Phys Act Health 2008;5(2):308–18.
55. Macko RF, Smith GV, Dobrovolny CL, et al. Treadmill training improves fitness reserve in chronic stroke patients. Arch Phys Med Rehabil 2001;82(7):879–84.
56. Michael K, Macko RF. Ambulatory activity intensity profiles, fitness, and fatigue in chronic stroke. Top Stroke Rehabil 2007;14(2):5–12.
57. Donovan K, Lord SE, McNaughton HK, et al. Mobility beyond the clinic: the effect of environment on gait and its measurement in community-ambulant stroke survivors. Clin Rehabil 2008;22(6):556–63.
58. Gebruers N, Vanroy C, Truijen S, et al. Monitoring of physical activity after stroke: a systematic review of accelerometry-based measures. Arch Phys Med Rehabil 2010;91(2):288–97.
59. Lord SE, Rochester L, Weatherall M, et al. The effect of environment and task on gait parameters after stroke: a randomized comparison of measurement conditions. Arch Phys Med Rehabil 2006;87(7):967–73.
60. Brauer SG, Morris ME. Can people with Parkinson's disease improve dual tasking when walking? Gait Posture 2010;31(2):229–33.
61. Lord SE, McPherson K, McNaughton HK, et al. Community ambulation after stroke: how important and obtainable is it and what measures appear predictive? Arch Phys Med Rehabil 2004;85(2):234–9.
62. Blennerhassett JM, Dite W, Ramage ER, et al. Changes in balance and walking from stroke rehabilitation to the community: a follow-up observational study. Arch Phys Med Rehabil 2012;93(10):1782–7.
63. Trigg R, Wood VA. The Subjective Index of Physical and Social Outcome (SIPSO): a new measure for use with stroke patients. Clin Rehabil 2000;14(3):288–99.
64. Wood-Dauphinee SL, Opzoomer MA, Williams JI, et al. Assessment of global function: the Reintegration to Normal Living Index. Arch Phys Med Rehabil 1988;69(8):583–90.
65. Bergner M, Bobbitt RA, Carter WB, et al. The Sickness Impact Profile: development and final revision of a health status measure. Med Care 1981;19(8):787–805.

66. Holbrook M, Skilbeck CE. An activities index for use with stroke patients. Age Ageing 1983;12(2):166–70.
67. Nouri FM, Lincoln NB. An extended activities of daily living scale for stroke patients. Clin Rehabil 1987;1(4):301–5.
68. Duncan PW, Wallace D, Lai SM, et al. The stroke impact scale version 2.0. Evaluation of reliability, validity, and sensitivity to change. Stroke 1999;30(10): 2131–40.
69. Movement Disorder Society Task Force on Rating Scales for Parkinson's Disease. The Unified Parkinson's Disease Rating Scale (UPDRS): status and recommendations. Mov Disord 2003;18(7):738–50.
70. Tulsky DS, Jette AM, Kisala PA, et al. Spinal cord injury-functional index: item banks to measure physical functioning in individuals with spinal cord injury. Arch Phys Med Rehabil 2012;93(10):1722–32.
71. Stucki G, Ewert T, Cieza A. Value and application of the ICF in rehabilitation medicine. Disabil Rehabil 2003;25(11–12):628–34.
72. Jette AM. Toward a common language for function, disability, and health. Phys Ther 2006;86(5):726–34.
73. Asano M, Miller WC, Eng JJ. Development and psychometric properties of the ambulatory self-confidence questionnaire. Gerontology 2007;53(6):373–81.
74. Shumway-Cook A, Patla A, Stewart AL, et al. Assessing environmentally determined mobility disability: self-report versus observed community mobility. J Am Geriatr Soc 2005;53(4):700–4.
75. Orendurff MS, Schoen JA, Bernatz GC, et al. How humans walk: bout duration, steps per bout, and rest duration. J Rehabil Res Dev 2008;45(7):1077–89.
76. Halstead LS. Longitudinal unobtrusive measurements in rehabilitation. Arch Phys Med Rehabil 1976;57(4):189–93.
77. Mudge S, Stott NS. Timed walking tests correlate with daily step activity in persons with stroke. Arch Phys Med Rehabil 2009;90(2):296–301.
78. Yarossi M, Franco B, Nolan KJ. StepWatch measures of community ambulation in individuals with hemiplegia following stroke. Archives of Physical Medicine and Rehabilitation–ACRM/ASNR Annual Conference 2011;92(10):1720.
79. Roos MA, Rudolph KS, Reisman DS. The structure of walking activity in people after stroke compared with older adults without disability: a cross-sectional study. Phys Ther 2012;92(9):1141–7.
80. Cavanaugh JT, Ellis TD, Earhart GM, et al. Capturing ambulatory activity decline in Parkinson's disease. J Neurol Phys Ther 2012;36(2):51–7.
81. Saraf P, Rafferty MR, Moore JL, et al. Daily stepping in individuals with motor incomplete spinal cord injury. Phys Ther 2010;90(2):224–35.
82. van de Port IG, Kwakkel G, Lindeman E. Community ambulation in patients with chronic stroke: how is it related to gait speed? J Rehabil Med 2008;40(1):23–7.

Gait Analysis for Poststroke Rehabilitation

The Relevance of Biomechanical Analysis and the Impact of Gait Speed

Sylvie Nadeau, PT, PhD[a,b,*], Martina Betschart, PT, MSc[a,b],
Francois Bethoux, MD[c]

KEYWORDS

- Gait analysis • Stroke • Ground reaction forces • Gait training • Rehabilitation

KEY POINTS

- Analysis of the time-distance parameters in patients who have had strokes reveals that they walk more slowly than healthy age-matched subjects. Reduced gait speed is combined with deviations in stride and step length, and/or lateral foot placement.
- Motion analysis shows that the angular excursion profiles of lower extremity joints are similar to those of healthy individuals, but the amplitude of peak values is reduced in subjects who have had strokes.
- Kinetic measurements (including the analysis of ground reaction forces) shows that patients who have had strokes have an asymmetric gait pattern and a decrease in peak moments and powers on the hemiparetic side. The hip flexors contribute more than the plantarflexors to energy generation while walking, contrary to what is observed in healthy individuals walking at self-selected speed.

INTRODUCTION

Stroke remains a major public health problem in many countries, afflicting nearly 15 million people worldwide each year (World Health Organization; http://www.strokecenter.org/patients/about-stroke/stroke-statistics/). Of this number, 5 million die and another 5 million are permanently disabled. Although the magnitude of the health care resources used to rehabilitate stroke survivors is considerable, many

[a] Pathokinesiology Laboratory, Centre for Interdisciplinary Research in Rehabilitation of Greater Montreal (CRIR), Institut de réadaptation Gingras-Lindsay-de-Montréal and School of Rehabilitation, University of Montreal, 6300 Avenue Darlington, Montreal, Quebec H3S 2J4, Canada; [b] The Multidisciplinary SensoriMotor Rehabilitation Research Team, Quebec, Canada; [c] The Mellen Center for Multiple Sclerosis Treatment and Research, The Cleveland Clinic Foundation, 9500 Euclid Avenue/Desk U10, Cleveland, OH 44195, USA
* Corresponding author.
E-mail address: sylvie.nadeau@umontreal.ca

Phys Med Rehabil Clin N Am 24 (2013) 265–276
http://dx.doi.org/10.1016/j.pmr.2012.11.007
1047-9651/13/$ – see front matter © 2013 Elsevier Inc. All rights reserved.

stroke victims continue to live with significant locomotor impairments. Moreover, the successful recovery of gait after stroke continues to be a day-to-day challenge for patients and for rehabilitation specialists.

The effects of gait training in individuals who have had strokes are characterized by large confidence intervals for mean differences in gait parameters at the end of training.[1] This variable response to training has been attributed to the heterogeneity of the participants, as well as to the variability in the response to a given intervention. Moreover, although gait patterns are generally asymmetrical,[2] large between-individual gait pattern differences exist,[3–5] suggesting the need for a more individualized approach to therapy based on personalized gait pattern indicators and sensorimotor impairments.

Physicians and clinicians trained to care for patients with central neurologic conditions frequently carry out an observational gait assessment to characterize their patients' specific gait dysfunctions in the context of routine clinical practice. The use of the naked eye or video images for gait analysis provides useful information to guide locomotor training. Many visual gait analysis rating scales, such as the Rancho Los Amigos System,[6–8] the Wisconsin Gait Scale (WGS), the Gait Assessment and Intervention Tool (GAIT),[9] and the Rivermead Visual Gait Assessment (RVGA), enable clinicians to describe pathologic gait deviations by body segments. However, as mentioned in a previous publication, the problem with observational gait assessment is its subjectivity[10] and the lack of information on its psychometric properties (validity, reliability, responsiveness, and specificity). There needs to be more studies such as the one published by McGinley and colleagues[11] (2006) to determine a reasonable threshold of visual detection, and to demonstrate the clinicians' ability to accurately judge gait deviations in real-time observations. These investigators showed that, in a clearly defined task and with a single parameter to judge, such as push-off of the plantarflexors, physical therapists were able to rate the gait deviation accurately.

A three-dimensional (3D) gait laboratory designed for performing a complete biomechanical gait analysis (including spatiotemporal measurements, kinematics, kinetics, and electromyographic data) allows the quantification of the locomotor pattern of a person with neurologic impairments after stroke.[12] The analysis identifies gait deficits and adaptive strategies, which, when combined with a neurologic assessment, can guide clinicians toward the causes of deviations and help them design the best and most effective locomotor training strategy for their patients. In addition, gait analysis allows the documentation of changes in relative effort, balance, and gait parameter variability (repeatability). Further, when used during a gait training session, this laboratory assessment can determine whether a patient is responding to the chosen intervention. Instrumented gait analysis remains the gold standard for gait assessment, although it can be argued that a complete biomechanical gait analysis with electromyography requires expensive equipment, time, and qualified personnel to prepare patients for the assessment, and to collect and interpret the data.

This article summarizes the process of gait analysis and the most important gait parameters and deviations in individuals who have had strokes, with specific emphasis on the effects of gait speed and the importance of ground reaction forces (GRFs).

Spatiotemporal Parameters

In the clinic, in the absence of appropriate equipment, it is difficult to measure the duration of each phase of the gait cycle, and to calculate which proportion of the cycle they represent. The use of instrumented surfaces, or sensors under the patient's feet, allows the capture of spatiotemporal parameters. The stride characteristics are recorded with 3 sensors located on the sole of the subject's shoe (heel, metatarsal heads, and big toe). The spatiotemporal parameters of gait can also be measured using a pressure-sensitive mat, such as the GAITRite mat (CIR Systems, Clifton, NJ). The GAITRite mat is a surface that contains a grid of sensors. The system records footfalls and also the time of activation/deactivation in relation to the location of activated sensors. Data are sampled and stored on a computer that calculates spatial and temporal parameters using dedicated software. The output from the GAITRite software is exported as a text file for further calculations. Gait symmetry measures (temporal and spatial) are calculated as ratios of the spatiotemporal values from the left and right lower limbs. In addition to symmetry parameters, gait velocity, cadence, stride length, step length, cycle time, and single and double support times can be measured. The concurrent validity and reliability of the GAITRite system has been established.[13,14]

The spontaneous gait speed of hemiparetic individuals is decreased, and is usually between 0.08 m/s and 1.05 m/s, compared with an average gait speed of 1.0 to 1.5 m/s in healthy individuals.[15–17] Gait speed is influenced by stride length and cadence (number of steps/min).[15,16,18] In healthy individuals, the spontaneous cadence is 115 steps/min on average,[19] whereas it can be markedly decreased after a stroke: between 27.9 and 47.2 steps/min according to Bohannon[20] and 57 steps/min according to Brandstater and colleagues,[21] even in subjects with good motor recovery. Step and stride length are also reduced after a stroke, and this further contributes to decreasing walking speed. Balasubramanian and colleagues[22] showed that step length asymmetry is closely linked to a lack of propulsive force generation on the paretic side. In a recent study, the same investigators[23] showed that not only front and back foot placement but also lateral foot placement relative to the pelvis in hemiparetic subjects differs from that of healthy subjects, depending on the walking speed. The results show that lateral asymmetry (the difference in foot position relative to the pelvis) is significantly related to the percentage of body weight supported by the paretic limb. The investigators recommend quantifying foot position relative to the pelvis in addition to step length.

Changes in walking speed, cadence, and step (or stride) length are associated with changes in the durations and proportions of the phases of the gait cycle. At spontaneous walking speed, a normal gait cycle, corresponding with the period between two successive strikes of the same foot (most often heel strike), has an average duration of 0.8 to 1.2 seconds.[24] In a hemiparetic individual walking more slowly, the cycle time increases to 1.8[25] to 2.22 seconds.[26] To analyze gait and allow a comparison between individuals, the gait cycle must be normalized between 0% and 100% and divided into a stance phase and a swing phase. In the healthy adult, the stance phase represents 60% to 62% of the gait cycle on average, whereas the swing phase represents 38% to 40%.[19] The stance phase is subdivided into a single support phase (about 40% of the gait cycle) and two double support phases (20%–24% of the gait cycle). The swing phase is subdivided into an initial, middle, and final phase. The stance phase in stroke survivors represents a greater part of the gait cycle compared with healthy individuals, both on the nonparetic side and on the paretic side, but the difference is more pronounced on the paretic side. In addition, the double support time is increased in hemiparetic individuals,[18,27] representing 52 ± 17% of the gait cycle according to Roth and colleagues.[26] These changes are caused in part by the decrease in walking speed.[28] The swing phase seems to be most affected (reduced) in individuals with slow or very slow walking speed (0.72–2.18 seconds or 25%–54% of the gait cycle, compared with 0.4 seconds and 40% of the gait cycle in healthy individuals).[29] Some investigators report that the swing phase is a determining phase of the gait cycle, and that its improvement leads to improved gait symmetry.[28,30] However, spatiotemporal parameters allow the characterization of the gait of hemiparetic individuals, but, used alone, they do not allow the cause of the observed deviations to be inferred.

Kinematics

Kinematics describe body motions independently from the internal and external forces that cause them. They are described in the 3 planes of space and include linear and angular motions, velocities, and accelerations. 3D kinematic gait parameters can be measured with passive systems such as the Vicon system (Vicon, Oxford, UK) or the ELITE optoelectronic system (BTS spa, Milano, Italy) with 6 cameras. This technology uses markers that reflect projected light (retroreflective markers). After the subjects have been instrumented with the markers (usually clusters of markers attached to rigid bodies on standard and specific anatomic landmarks), 3D gait data are collected with infrared cameras. Then the spatial location of each circular reflective marker placed on the skin is determined by identifying (automatically or by user input) the bright spots on the screen that belong to each physical marker. Reflective marker systems require time to digitize the x, y, and z coordinates and mathematical models to reconstruct the coordinates of the markers. The markers have to be identified and potential merging of markers in various camera views places limitations on how close to each other the markers may be placed. Passive markers are less constraining for the subject (the subject is not tethered to wires), but they require a more intelligent data processing system. Other advantages of passive markers include ease of attachment to the body segments, which allows the subject under analysis maximum freedom of movement, and, at least theoretically, the use of a potentially unlimited number of markers. In general, passive marker systems require the collection of calibration data before recording the position of the markers placed on a given segment. In contrast, active marker systems (**Fig. 1**), such as the Optotrak system (Northern Digital Inc, Waterloo, Ontario, Canada), use light-emitting diode (LED) markers that are pulsed sequentially, so the system automatically knows the identification of each marker. Only 1 LED is turned on at any instant in time. The cameras then uniquely identify the instant spatial location of that marker. The marker coordinates are automatically identified. The main advantage of active markers is their easier labeling. Marker tracking is not a problem and merging markers cannot occur with these systems, thus the markers can be placed close to each other. Overall, active marker systems exhibit excellent accuracy. Drawbacks include that they require wires to be attached to each marker, and that there is no video image to concomitantly view or record the subject's movements (see **Fig. 1**).

The markers are placed on relevant body segments (feet, lower legs, thighs, pelvis), as shown in **Fig. 1**. An anthropometric model is used to represent the subject's characteristics. The proximal, distal, and largest circumference of each limb segment can be measured, along with the subject's body weight, to model the segment geometry and the position of the segment's center of mass and mass, based on anthropometric references such as those published by Winter.[31] Inertia moments are also computed from the length, diameters, and mass of the limb segments.[32] To obtain true 3D motion analysis, each group of 3 markers (which create a plane passing through the segment) should be continuously recorded (usually around 60 Hz) while the subject walks, and joint centers as well as angles (eg, Euler) must be defined. Kinematic data are

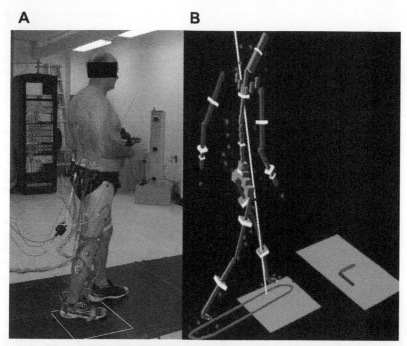

Fig. 1. (*A*) Participant equipped with active markers recorded with an Optotrak system. Electromyography electrodes are also shown on the gastrocnemius and lateral hamstring. (*B*) A modeled participant during walking. The rigid body segments, light–emitting diodes, instrumented surfaces, reaction force vector underneath the left foot, and global center of pressure and center of mass are observable. The transverse view of the contour of the base of support associated to the foot contact with the ground is also represented.

filtered and software is used to calculate the relative angles (eg, Euler, Cardanic). The local x, y, and z axes correspond with the abduction-adduction, longitudinal rotation, and flexion-extension axes for the hip and knee joints, whereas at the ankle they corresponded with the eversion-inversion, transverse rotation, and dorsiflexion-plantarflexion axes, respectively.

This article only discusses angular motions in the plane sagittal to the lower extremities. After a stroke, the angular excursion profiles for lower extremity joints are similar to those of healthy individuals. However, the occurrence and amplitude of peak values differ from the norms, and the difference is more noticeable as the walking speed deviates from that of healthy individuals,[2] as shown in **Fig. 2**. At the early stance phase, published studies report a flat foot strike, associated with increased knee flexion and decreased hip flexion. A decrease in plantarflexion and hip extension subsequently brings the knee into hyperextension. During the swing phase, in addition to decreased knee flexion, circumduction of the leg or exaggerated hip flexion allows adequate foot clearance.[16,33] Kinematic changes are also observed on the intact side, with increased knee flexion during swing phase and decreased knee extension during stance phase. However, these changes are less pronounced than those observed on the affected side.[2,5,16] Kinematic values vary among individuals with hemiparesis, therefore the data should be analyzed with caution.[2] It is therefore important to examine in detail the angular displacements in each patient, to assess deviations and to establish an individualized treatment plan.

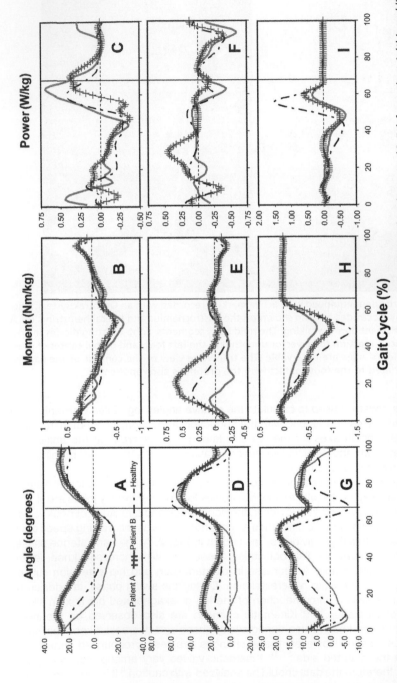

Fig. 2. Angle profiles at the hip (*A*), knee (*D*), and ankle (*G*), and corresponding moments (*B*, *E*, *H*) and powers (*C*, *F*, *I*) for patient A (*thin red line*) and patient B (*thick blue line*). The dotted lines refer to healthy subjects walking at matched cadences (85 steps/min). The gait speeds are 0.78, 0.85, and 0.92 (±0.10) m/s for patient A, patient B, and healthy subjects respectively. The gait cycle is normalized to 100% and the data are for the paretic side for the patients and the dominant side for the healthy group.

Kinetics

Kinetics refer to the internal and external forces resulting in the specific movement pattern observed.[34] Moments and powers are obtained from measurements of the GRFs, combined with kinematic data in an inverted dynamic model at each 1% interval of the gait cycle.[34] During gait, the net moment of a joint equals the sum of the active moment produced by muscle contraction and the passive moment associated with the joint's noncontractile structures (ie, capsule and connective tissues). Maximum values for moments and powers increase with walking speed. Similar to kinematic variables, the net positive moment and power of the hip, knee, and ankle on the affected side have a profile comparable with that of healthy individuals, but the amplitude is often decreased,[2,5,35] as shown in **Fig. 2**. At the hip, the energy generated by the extensors at the beginning of the gait cycle (H1) can be null, less or higher than that of healthy individuals (approximately 0.2 W/kg), depending on the study.[2,5] The energy generation from the hip flexors (approximately 0.5 W/kg) remains present in hemiparetic individuals, but tends to decrease as the walking speed decreases.[2,5] At the ankle, the net positive power (approximately 0.9 W/kg) generated by the concentric contraction of the plantar-flexors during the push-off phase (A2) still contributes to energy generation, but to a lesser degree, as shown by Morita and colleagues.[36] Moreover, the energy generation from the plantarflexors is absent in hemiparetic individuals who walk at a very low speed ($\leq$0.25 m/s).[2] Therefore, the hip flexors contribute more than the plantarflexors to energy generation while walking, contrary to what is observed in healthy individuals walking at self-selected speeds.[33] On the nonaffected side, the same trends are observed; however, the net moment and power, although still less than normal values, are greater compared with the affected side.[2,5] The ratio of the energy produced by muscles on the nonaffected side compared with the affected side is around 60:40, and remains similar at various degrees of walking capacity.[2,5]

Researchers recently estimated the level of effort for key muscle groups on both sides, in healthy and hemiparetic individuals. Subjects in the stroke group showed a greater level of effort (45%–78%) than able-bodied subjects matched for cadence (24%–63%). For both groups, the level of effort was similar between sides and increased with cadence. At self-selected cadence, the plantarflexors showed greater relative effort values, whereas, at maximal cadence, levels of effort for all muscles were equivalent. The investigators concluded that, for a similar cadence, the levels of effort of hemiparetic individuals were greater than those of able-bodied individuals.[37,38] As with able-bodied individuals, community-walker hemiparetic individuals had effort values that increased significantly with speed, with the hip muscles presenting the largest gain. However, the effort values of these hemiparetic individuals were greater than those of healthy individuals matched for cadence. These results also suggested that the hemiparetic partici-pants spontaneously decreased their self-selected speed to keep their level of effort similar to that observed in able-bodied individuals walking at self-selected speed.[37,38]

GRFs and Walking Speed

The GRF is represented by 3 components that correspond with the forces the human body exerts to the ground during walking (**Fig. 3**). In the analysis of gait pattern, the main task is the forward propulsion of the body's center of mass (COM), which can be analyzed by capturing the anterior-posterior force during

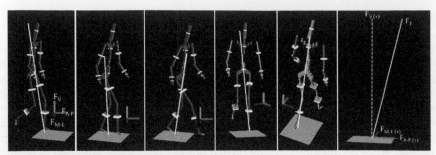

Fig. 3. GRF during walking. Anteroposterior force (F_{A-P}), mediolateral force (F_{M-L}), vertical force (F_V), and total force (F_T). Positive directions are also shown.

walking.[39] The vertical GRF (V-GRF) is related to the weight support of the acting/moving subject.[40] There is also a mediolateral force. The mediolateral acceleration of the COM is equal to the total mediolateral GRF (ML-GRF) divided by the body mass.[41] These 3 forces are all related to stance duration and body mass.[3,40,42] The GRF analysis has been used as a method to assess the gait pattern of stroke survivors.[2,3,5,35,36,39,40,42,43]

Among the components of the GRF, the vertical force is the most important, and its intensity exceeds that of body weight. The curve is characterized by 2 peaks (**Fig. 4**). At heel strike, there is a rapid increase in force, and the first peak is quickly reached. Then a progressive decrease is observed, down to a minimum that corresponds with unipodal stance. A subsequent increase leads to the second peak, at push-off. The anterior-posterior force results from horizontal linear accelerations, and is approximately 10 times less than the vertical force. It reflects the deceleration (negative values) and the propulsion (positive values) of the body during stance phase. The second horizontal force (mediolateral) is of low intensity. This force represents the acceleration of body segments in the frontal plane, in relation to lateral body movements. During walking, this force is mainly negative, which means that it is directed toward the center of the body. As with moments and powers, the intensity of these forces is influenced by the individual's body mass and by the cadence and gait speed. Anteroposterior GRFs allow the contribution of the paretic lower limb to forward body propulsion while walking to be determined. Bowden and colleagues[43] reported that, at a gait speed of 1.2 m/s, the area under the curve (AUC) is similar for all forces. However, when the gait speed is between 0.44 and 0.6 m/s, the AUCs were asymmetrical, and showed decreased propulsion in the paretic limb and increased propulsion in the nonparetic limb. In **Fig. 4**, mean GRF profiles clearly reveal a significant difference in the stance phase percentage between sides. The gait speed modifies the moment of the gait cycle where the peak GRF values occur. The asymmetry between sides is greater for the propulsive force (AP-P2) than for the braking force (AP-P1) and the latter is not modified by speed. For the Vertical force (V), at both speeds, the asymmetry is greater at the end of the stance phase (V-P3) than at the beginning. V-P1 and V-P2 values are often greater on the affected side (A) than on the UA side. Asymmetry increased with speed only for the third peak (V-P3). The Medio-Lateral force (ML) reveals between sides asymmetry of the negative component (ML-P2) and an increase is observed with gait speed, with values being higher on the A side. Overall the GRF differ from those of healthy subjects and the differences between sides can be appreciated both at self-selected and fast speeds.

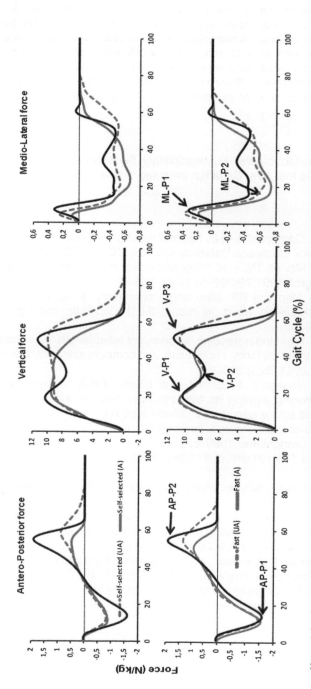

Fig. 4. Unaffected (UA) and affected (A) GRF mean profiles in individuals with hemiparesis walking at self-selected (*red lines*) and fast (*blue lines*) speeds. The full dark lines refer to healthy subjects walking at self-selected speed (dominant side). The peaks for each GRF component are identified. Average (standard deviation) gait speed was as follows: patients who have had strokes (n = 35), self-selected speed 0.72 (0.26) m/s, fast speed1.08 (0.46) m/s. Healthy controls (n = 14), self-selected speed used as reference, 1.26 (0.19) m/s (cadence 106 [11.5] steps/min, stride length 1.42 (0.11) m). AP, anteroposterior force; AP-P1, braking force (negative peak); AP-P2, propulsive force (positive peak); ML, mediolateral force; ML-P1, maximum peak at initial stance (lateral force); ML-P2, minimum peak (medial force); V, vertical force; V-P1, first maximum peak; V-P2, minimum peak between first and second maximum peaks; V-P3, second maximum peak.

SUMMARY

The hemiparetic gait after stroke is characterized by a reduced walking speed, an asymmetric gait pattern, and a decrease in peak moments and powers on the hemiparetic side. Most studies have analyzed walking in the sagittal plane. Some characteristics are common between patients, but significant differences in gait pattern may occur between hemiparetic individuals, even if their walking speeds are comparable. As with the other gait parameters, GRFs are helpful in interpreting the gait pattern deviations of patients after stroke as well as other neurologic populations.

ACKNOWLEDGMENTS

This work was supported by the Multidisciplinary Sensorimotor Rehabilitation Research Team (Strategic Initiative, Canadian Institutes of Health Research [CIHR]).

REFERENCES

1. Moseley AM, Stark A, Cameron ID, et al. Treadmill training and body weight support for walking after stroke. Cochrane Database Syst Rev 2005;(4):CD002840.
2. Olney SJ, Griffin MP, Monga TN, et al. "Work and power in gait of stroke patients". Arch Phys Med Rehabil 1991;72:309–14.
3. Allen JL, Kautz SA, Neptune RR. Step length asymmetry is representative of compensatory mechanisms used in post-stroke hemiparetic walking. Gait Posture 2011;33:538–43.
4. Roerdink M, Beek PJ. Understanding inconsistent step-length asymmetries across hemiplegic stroke patients: impairments and compensatory gait. Neurorehabil Neural Repair 2011;25(3):253–8.
5. Teixeira-Salmela LF, Nadeau S, McBride I, et al. Effects of muscle strengthening and physical conditioning training on temporal, kinematic and kinetic variables during gait in chronic stroke survivors. J Rehabil Med 2001;33(2):53–60.
6. Olsson EC. Methods of studying gait. In: Smidt GL, editor. Gait in rehabilitation. New York: Churchill Livingstone; 1990. p. 2143.
7. Perry J. Gait analysis. Normal and pathological function. Thorofare (NJ): SLACK; 1992.
8. Perry J, Burnfield JM. Gait analysis: normal and pathological function. 2e edition. Thorofare (NJ): SLACK; 2010.
9. Daly JJ, Nethery J, McCabe JP, et al. Development and testing of the Gait Assessment and Intervention Tool (G.A.I.T.): a measure of coordinated gait components. J Neurosci Methods 2009;178(2):334–9.
10. Toro B, Nester C, Farren P. A review of observational gait assessment in clinical practice [Review]. Physiother Theor Pract 2003;19(3):137–49.
11. McGinley JL, Goldie PA, Greenwood KM, et al. Accuracy and reliability of observational gait analysis data: judgments of push-off in gait after stroke. Phys Ther 2003;83(2):146–60.
12. Nadeau S, Duclos C, Bouyer L, et al. Guiding task-oriented gait training after stroke or spinal cord injury (SCI) by means of a biomechanical gait analysis. In: Green AM, Chapman CE, Kalaskav J, et al, editors. Progress in brain research. Amsterdam: 2011. p. 161–80.
13. McDonough AL, Batavia M, Chen FC, et al. The validity and reliability of the GAITRite system's measurements: a preliminary evaluation. Arch Phys Med Rehabil 2001;82:419–25.

14. Bilney B, Morris M, Webster K. Concurrent related validity of the GAITRite walkway system for quantification of the spatial and temporal parameters of gait. Gait Posture 2003;17:68–74, 29,30.

15. Beaman CB, Peterson CL, Neptune RR, et al. Differences in self-selected and fastest-comfortable walking in post-stroke hemiparetic persons [Research Support, N.I.H., Extramural Research Support, U.S. Government, Non-P.H.S.]. Gait Posture 2010;31(3):311–6.

16. Olney SJ, Richards C. Hemiparetic gait following stroke. Part I. Characteristics. Gait Posture 1996;4:136–48.

17. Shiavi R, Bugle HJ, Limbird T. Electromyographic gait assessment, part 1: adult EMG profiles and walking speed. J Rehabil Res Dev 1987;24(2):13–23.

18. Von Schroeder HP, Coutts RD, Lyden PD, et al. Gait parameters following stroke: a practical assessment. J Rehabil Res Dev 1995;32(1):25–31.

19. Rose J, Gamble JG, Inman VT. Human walking. Philadelphia: Lippincott Williams and Wilkins; 2006.

20. Bohannon RW. Selected determinants of ambulatory capacity in patients with hemiplegia. Clin Rehabil 1989;3:47–53.

21. Brandstater ME, de Bruin H, Gowland C, et al. Hemiplegic gait: analysis of temporal variables. Arch Phys Med Rehabil 1983;64(12):583–7.

22. Balasubramanian CK, Bowden MG, Neptune RR, et al. Relationship between step length asymmetry and walking performance in subjects with chronic hemiparesis. Arch Phys Med Rehabil 2007;88(1):43–9.

23. Balasubramanian CK, Neptune RR, Kautz SA. Foot placement in a body reference frame during walking and its relationship to hemiparetic walking performance. Clin Biomech 2010;25(5):483–90.

24. Craik RL, Oatis CA. Gait analysis: theory and applications. St Louis (MO): Mosby-Year Book; 1995.

25. Ada L, Vattanasilp W, O'Dwyer NJ, et al. Does spasticity contribute to walking dysfunction after stroke? J Neurol Neurosurg Psychiatry 1998;64:628–35.

26. Roth EJ, Merbitz C, Mroczek K, et al. Hemiplegic gait: relationships between walking speed and other temporal parameters. Am J Phys Med Rehabil 1997; 76(2):128–33.

27. Sullivan KJ, Mulroy S, SA K. Walking recovery and rehabilitation after stroke. In: Stein Z, Harvey R, Macko R, et al, editors. Stroke recovery and rehabilitation. New York: Demos Medical Publishing; 2009. p. 323–42.

28. Patterson KK, Gage WH, Brooks D, et al. Evaluation of gait symmetry after stroke: a comparison of current methods and recommendations for standardization [Comparative Study, Research Support, Non-U.S. Government]. Gait Posture 2010;31(2):241–6.

29. De Quervain IA, Simon SR, Leurgans S, et al. Gait pattern in the early recovery period after stroke [Research Support, Non-U.S. Government Research Support, U.S. Government, P.H.S.]. J Bone Joint Surg Am 1996;78(10):1506–14.

30. Dimitrijevic MR, Faganel J, Sherwood AM, et al. Activation of paralysed leg flexors and extensors during gait in patients after stroke. Scand J Rehabil Med 1981;13(5):109–15.

31. Winter DA. Biomechanics and motor control of human movement. 2nd edition. New York: Wiley-Interscience; 1990.

32. Pavol MJ, Owings TM, Grabiner MD. Body segment inertial parameter estimation for the general population of older adults. J Biomech 2002;35(5):707–12.

33. Nadeau S, Gravel D, Olney SJ. Determinants, limiting factors and compensatory strategies in gait. Crit Rev Phys Rehabil Med 2001;13(1):1–24.

34. Winter DA. The biomechanics and motor control of human gait: normal, elderly and pathological. Waterloo (Canada): University of Waterloo Press; 1991.
35. Parvataneni K, Olney SJ, Brouwer B. Changes in muscle group work associated with changes in gait speed of persons with stroke. Clin Biomech 2007;22(7): 813–20.
36. Morita S, Yamamoto H, Furuya K. Gait analysis of hemiplegic patients by measurement of ground reaction force. Scand J Rehabil Med 1995;27(1):37–42.
37. Milot MH, Nadeau S, Gravel D, et al. Bilateral level of effort of the plantar flexors, hip flexors, and extensors during gait in hemiparetic and healthy individuals. Stroke 2006;37:2070–5.
38. Milot MH, Nadeau S, Gravel D. Muscular utilization of the plantarflexors, hip flexors and extensor muscles in persons with hemiparesis walking at self-selected and maximal speeds. J Electromyogr Kinesiol 2007;17:184–93.
39. Peterson CL, Cheng J, Kautz SA, et al. Leg extension is an important predictor of paretic leg propulsion in hemiparetic walking. Gait Posture 2010;32(4):451–6.
40. Kesar TM, Binder-Macleod SA, Hicks GE, et al. Minimal detectable change for gait variables collected during treadmill walking in individuals post-stroke. Gait Posture 2011;33(2):314–7.
41. Davis RB, Kaufman KR. Kinetics of normal walking. In: Rose J, Gamble JG, editors. Human walking. 3rd edition. Philadelphia: Lippincott Williams & Wilkins; 2006. p. 53–76.
42. John CT, Seth A, Schwartz MH, et al. Contributions of muscles to mediolateral ground reaction force over a range of walking speeds. J Biomech 2012;45(14): 2438–43.
43. Bowden MG, Balasubramanian CK, Neptune RR, et al. Anterior-posterior ground reaction forces as a measure of paretic leg contribution in hemiparetic walking. Stroke 2006;37(3):872–6.

Rehabilitation of Ambulatory Limitations

Lara A. Pilutti, PhD[a], Audrey L. Hicks, PhD[b],*

KEYWORDS

- Ambulation • Rehabilitation • Walking

KEY POINTS

- A variety of tools and techniques are available for the rehabilitation of ambulatory impairments in adults with central neurologic disorders.
- These strategies can be described as traditional and nontraditional.
- Each strategy has particular advantages and disadvantages with respect to feasibility, cost effectiveness, accessibility, and training specificity.
- The various rehabilitation strategies should be considered complementary rather than exclusive.
- Rehabilitation strategies should be selected using an individualized approach.

INTRODUCTION

Rehabilitation has been defined by the World Health Organization as "a proactive and goal-oriented activity to restore function and/or to maximize remaining function to bring about the highest possible level of independence, physically, psychologically, socially and economically."[1] The rehabilitation process ideally involves a multidisciplinary team of professionals to promote recovery in physical, psychological, and social domains.[1] Rehabilitation represents a particularly important strategy for the treatment of ambulatory limitations in adults who have central neurologic disorders. For certain neurologic populations, rehabilitation strategies may be the only effective mode of therapy to improve or maintain functional abilities. Deficits contributing to ambulatory limitations in adults with central neurologic disorders commonly include impaired walking speed and spatial and temporal parameters of gait, balance, lower extremity strength, and tone (spasticity)[2–8]; consequently, these targets are often the focus of ambulatory rehabilitation strategies. Individuals with neurologic diseases

Disclosure statement: The authors declare no conflicts of interest.
[a] Department of Kinesiology and Community Health, University of Illinois at Urbana-Champaign, 906 South Goodwin Avenue, Urbana, IL 61801, USA; [b] Department of Kinesiology, McMaster University, 1280 Main Street West, Hamilton, Ontario L8S 4K1, Canada
* Corresponding author.
E-mail address: hicksal@mcmaster.ca

Phys Med Rehabil Clin N Am 24 (2013) 277–290
http://dx.doi.org/10.1016/j.pmr.2012.11.008
1047-9651/13/$ – see front matter © 2013 Elsevier Inc. All rights reserved.

have unique clinical presentations and courses, and, as such, rehabilitation strategies should be prescribed based on the specific needs and deficits experienced by each patient.

Despite the importance of ambulatory rehabilitation for individuals with central neurologic disorders, there are several limitations of the current literature in this field. Common limitations include small sample sizes, lack of appropriate controls, substantial patient heterogeneity, lack of long-term interventions and follow-up, and inconsistent or insufficient outcomes for evaluating ambulation in individuals with neurologic impairment. The assessment of ambulatory rehabilitation strategies has typically included outcomes of walking velocity, walking endurance, spatial and temporal gait parameters, or clinical examination.[3] Importantly, the inclusion of real-life measures of ambulation (ie, pedometers and accelerometers) and patient-reported experiences of walking impairment have been increasingly included as outcomes in the evaluation of ambulatory limitations.[3]

Several strategies are currently available for the rehabilitation of ambulatory limitations in adults with central neurologic disorders that can be described as traditional or nontraditional rehabilitation. In general, traditional rehabilitation strategies are those that involve passive or active movements or exercises, whereas nontraditional therapies involve the use of advanced therapeutic technologies or devices. This article describes and evaluates the most common traditional and nontraditional therapies available for ambulatory rehabilitation in adults with central nervous system (CNS) disorders such as stroke, spinal cord injury (SCI), multiple sclerosis (MS), and Parkinson's disease (PD). Traditional rehabilitation strategies that will be explored include exercise training and conventional gait training. Nontraditional rehabilitation strategies that will be explored include functional electrical stimulation (FES), recumbent stepper training, body weight–supported treadmill training (BWSTT), and the ZeroG overground gait and balance training system. The advantages, disadvantages, and applications of each of these rehabilitation modalities are discussed. Rehabilitation is also often used in conjunction with other interventions for ambulation (eg, fitting and training to the use of an assistive device or orthosis, medical or surgical treatments for spasticity). Such an approach is often considered standard of care or best practice, and, as a consequence, there is little evidence showing the specific benefits of rehabilitation strategies in terms of the overall efficacy, safety, and acceptability of other interventions. We will, therefore, mostly focus our review on the effects of rehabilitation techniques when used alone.

TRADITIONAL REHABILITATION IN ADULTS WITH CENTRAL NEUROLOGIC CONDITIONS
Exercise Training

Exercise training has been widely administered as a rehabilitation strategy in adults with CNS disorders including stroke, SCI, MS, and PD.[9–17] The forms of exercise training that have been most commonly prescribed and that will be considered in this article include aerobic training and progressive resistance training, either alone or in combination. Traditional aerobic exercise training modalities used for individuals with neurologic diseases include treadmill walking, leg cycling ergometry, arm ergometry, and aquatic exercise. Resistance training regimes typically include weight machines, free weights, body weight exercises, cable pulleys, or elastic bands. Both of these exercise forms have been used successfully in the MS population to improve ambulatory outcomes. For example, 8 weeks of leg cycling ergometry (60 minutes, 3 sessions per week) at a moderate-to-strong intensity resulted in significant improvements in aerobic capacity, walking speed, and walking endurance in adults with MS.[18] Similarly, 12 weeks of lower extremity progressive resistance training resulted in lower limb strength gains and improved walking speed, endurance, and functional task performance in patients with MS.[19]

Traditional aerobic and resistance exercise can also be combined or enhanced with other techniques, such as biofeedback. For instance, biofeedback cycling provides patients with visual information regarding input from each individual leg allowing for the monitoring and correction of cycling asymmetries during training.[20,21] Correcting cycling asymmetries during exercise may translate into improvements in ambulation. Using this type of intervention, 6 sessions of leg pedaling exercise with biofeedback resulted in improved cycling asymmetry and improvement in walking speed and gait asymmetry in a case series of 3 chronic stroke patients.[20]

Physiologic deconditioning, or the loss of aerobic capacity and muscular strength, is common among adults with neurologic diseases.[22–27] This loss of physical fitness may, in turn, limit ambulatory capacity. Correctly prescribed exercise training is expected to improve aerobic endurance and muscular strength. As described in the aforementioned training studies,[18,19] the training-induced improvements in aerobic and muscular performance may also translate into meaningful benefits on ambulation.

There are several advantages to exercise training as a rehabilitation strategy. Exercise training is cost effective compared with many other modalities and generally available in most community settings. A combined program of aerobic and resistance training may also result in several health and fitness benefits, such as improved bone health, body composition, and comorbid disease risk profile.[28] The disadvantage of this modality is that it is generally not task specific to ambulation, with the exception of treadmill walking. Exercise training, however, may be used in combination with other task-specific rehabilitation techniques to improve cardiovascular endurance and muscular capacity, which may act synergistically to improve ambulation. Finally, for individuals with severe mobility limitations, traditional aerobic and resistance training equipment is often not physically accessible.

Conventional Gait Training

Conventional gait training is one of the most commonly used forms of rehabilitation for adults with CNS disorders and may include techniques such as overground walking and movement training; balance, coordination, and range of motion exercises; and active and passive stretching. The variety of techniques used in conventional gait training results in a targeted rehabilitation approach that can be specific to the gait impairments of each patient. Conventional gait training strategies are typically delivered by trained personnel, such as physical therapists, occupational therapists, or exercise professionals. With practice, some strategies may be undertaken outside of the clinical setting, particularly for patients who are capable of independent ambulation. Conventional gait training strategies have been used in patients with stroke, SCI, MS, and PD.[29–34] For example, a 6-week (3 sessions/week) physical or occupational therapist-supervised program involved practice of 10 walking-related tasks (ie, forward and backward walking, stepping, kicking, balancing, and sitting-to-standing transitions) in patients with chronic stroke.[31] Patients were further encouraged to practice at-home walking. This training program resulted in improvements in walking speed and distance compared with participants who were involved in seated upper extremity functional task training.

Conventional gait training techniques may also be supplemented with adjunct therapies, such as rhythmic auditory stimulation (RAS). RAS is described as a neurologic music therapy technique that targets gait dysfunction through the use of rhythmic timing cues.[35] RAS has been used in patients with several neurologic diseases and often in addition to conventional gait-training techniques.[35–37] For instance, patients with PD were involved in 6 weeks of stepping training with or without the use of RAS.[36] Compared with stepping practice alone, stepping with RAS resulted in superior improvements on functional gait and balance outcomes, and the effects were more long lasting after the intervention period. This highlights the importance of considering alternative and combined therapies when treating ambulatory impairments.

There are several important benefits to conventional gait training. Conventional gait training is task specific in that it allows patients the opportunity to practice walking and movement-related tasks. Unlike other strategies, training can be tailored to the specific gait deficits experienced by each patient because of the multifaceted rehabilitation approach. Conventional gait training is generally more cost effective than nontraditional rehabilitation strategies involving specialized equipment. Adjunct therapies such as RAS can also be incorporated to enhance outcomes. Unfortunately, the feasibility of conventional gait training may be limited for patients with severe mobility impairment, although likely not to the same extent as exercise training. This modality also requires expertise from specialized personnel, which may only be available at clinical rehabilitation centers.

NONTRADITIONAL REHABILITATION IN ADULTS WITH CENTRAL NEUROLOGIC CONDITIONS
Functional Electrical Stimulation

FES is a technique that delivers brief electrical pulses to muscles or peripheral nerves in patients with CNS disorders with the goal of improving function. To date, FES has been used in various populations, particularly in stroke survivors and individuals with SCI, to facilitate ambulatory function and improve muscle strength.[38–40] The earliest uses of FES in the stroke population was to improve or correct foot drop (through peroneal nerve stimulation),[41] but later studies tended to explore the broader utility of FES to improve specific aspects of walking performance in stroke survivors, such as gait kinematics, muscle spasticity, and muscle strength. There is good evidence that FES is effective in improving gait speed in individuals after stroke, although it may provide more of an orthotic as opposed to therapeutic benefit (ie, the improvements may not necessarily be maintained when the FES is removed).[42] The strongest evidence for a benefit of FES to improve ambulation after stroke is when it is combined with other gait retraining strategies.[40,43] In the SCI population, FES-assisted walking has been used as both an orthotic aid (for complete or incomplete paraplegics) and as a therapeutic modality to improve gait in people with incomplete SCI.[38] To date, FES-assisted walking therapy has not been found to be superior to other ambulatory training interventions (eg, BWSTT, overground walking training) in people with chronic incomplete SCI, although greater benefits may be seen with combined approaches.[44,45] Further information about the use of FES after stroke and SCI can be found elsewhere in this issue.

Potential advantages to FES-assisted walking training include the ability to promote active movement of limb segments (as opposed to immobilization of joints and limb segments with traditional orthoses), thereby, decreasing the risk of nonuse muscle atrophy and range of motion limitations, relative safety and ease of use, and the potential to promote CNS plasticity through repetitive afferent feedback from the muscle contraction and limb motion generated by the stimulation. However, limitations of FES-assisted walking training should also be considered. First, this rehabilitation technique can only be applied in individuals with intact lower motoneurons and viable peripheral nerves (and neuromuscular junctions) to the lower limb musculature. Second, clinically available systems of FES-assisted walking cannot stimulate the hip flexors directly; thus, any hip flexion during walking has to be initiated voluntarily by the patient. Third, the muscles stimulated through FES experience rapid fatigue because the larger-diameter (and more fatigable) nerve fibers are most easily stimulated by surface electrodes, which significantly limits the length of time that FES-assisted walking can be performed. Finally, the electrical current excites both motor and sensory nerves and may be painful to some individuals, especially those with preserved sensation.[38]

Recumbent Stepper Training

Recumbent stepper training allows patients to step against graded resistive forces from a supported seated position (**Fig. 1**). Coupled arm levers and foot pedals move in a bilateral reciprocal manner, which results in movement of the lower and upper extremities. The coupled upper and lower body training system allows for compensation of upper or lower extremity weakness in a self-driven manner in that all movement is patient initiated. Additional features of the recumbent stepper can include adjustable arm levers, rotating seat, large foot pedals with exterior edges, foot and arm strapping, and leg stabilizers, which make this piece of equipment accessible and adaptable for persons with varying degrees of disability. To date, the effects of recumbent stepper training in adults with neurologic diseases have only been examined by 2 research groups: one in patients with stroke[46] and the other in patients with PD.[47] Patients with PD who participated in 10–12 weeks of 3 weekly sessions (30 minutes per session) of recumbent stepper training experienced improvements in walking speed and step length, although there was no change in the severity of disability.[47] Further trials in a variety of neurologic disease populations are necessary to determine the potential of recumbent stepper training as a tool for the rehabilitation of ambulatory limitations.

Recumbent stepper training may target ambulatory deficits through several different mechanisms. The full-body aerobic training stimulus may result in improvements in aerobic and muscular performance, similar to traditional exercise training. In sedentary adults, recumbent stepper training has been found to improve peak aerobic capacity and strength and endurance of both upper and lower extremity muscles.[48] Improved aerobic endurance and muscle strength may, in turn, improve ambulatory

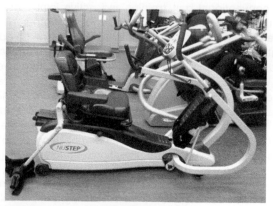

Fig. 1. Recumbent stepper training (Nustep, TRS 400, Ann Arbor, MI).

performance, although this requires further investigation in specific neurologic populations. The stepping motion of recumbent stepper training has also been shown to have a similar, although less complex, neuromuscular activation pattern to walking,[49] suggesting specificity of this training modality to ambulation; however, the joint kinematics of recumbent stepping are different than those involved in walking.

Compared with most nontraditional rehabilitation modalities, recumbent stepper training is cost effective and simple to operate. This modality could be easily implemented in community and home settings. The accessibility and adapted accessories available for this piece of equipment make it applicable to individuals with varying disability levels. The self-driven nature of the modality also allows for all work to be conducted by the patient rather than requiring substantial assistance from therapists or devices, likely resulting in greater overall effort by the patient. The main disadvantage of this system is that it is less specific to ambulation than other nontraditional rehabilitation techniques. The movement is also restricted to stepping and would not allow participants to practice other ambulatory movements, such as balancing or transferring tasks.

Body Weight–Supported Treadmill Training

BWSTT consists of a motorized treadmill with an overhead counterbalancing system attached to a supportive harness (**Fig. 2**). Using the support harness, patients are suspended over the treadmill with a certain amount of their body weight off-loaded by the counterbalancing system. This system allows patients with neurologic impairment and limited mobility to practice walking in an upright position without the risk of falling. The initial amount of body weight support required is selected to allow patients to maintain an upright torso and to prevent knee buckling while standing. When necessary, movement of the lower extremities can be facilitated through therapist assistance or robotic assistance. Typically, therapist-assisted training involves 2 trainers positioned one at each lower limb to guide the patient through the proper walking kinematics. An additional therapist can be positioned behind the patient to assist in weight shifting and stabilization when necessary. Robotic-assisted gait training involves the use of a motorized orthosis, which is attached to the patients' lower extremities. The gait orthosis assists patients in moving their lower limbs through proper gait cycle motions and is controlled by a computerized system. Studies of BWSTT have been conducted with patients with SCI, stroke, MS, and PD and have evaluated both therapist-assisted and robotic-assisted training regimes.[50–54] For example, patients with PD participated in 12 sessions (45 minutes per session) of robotic-assisted gait training or physiotherapy involving conventional gait training and active joint mobilization.[55] Robot-assisted gait training was superior to conventional physiotherapy on outcomes of walking speed, walking endurance, and some spatiotemporal gait parameters.

The main advantage of BWSTT is the task-specific nature of the training modality as a tool for the rehabilitation of ambulation. BWSTT is also an alternative for patients with severe disability who are unable to participate in traditional training modalities because of inaccessibility of the equipment. The use of robot assistance may also place less physical burden on the therapists and provide a more normal and consistent gait pattern.[56] Superiority of therapist-assisted or robotic-assisted treadmill training over traditional gait training, however, has not been established in patients with neurologic diseases.[57–59] Several limitations of this training modality exist. Although BWSTT may allow for the practice of walking specifically, it does not allow for the practice of other ambulatory movements that may also be important to activities of daily living. It has been suggested that restricting and controlling patients' gait patterns through therapist or robotic assistance may not allow for the opportunity to

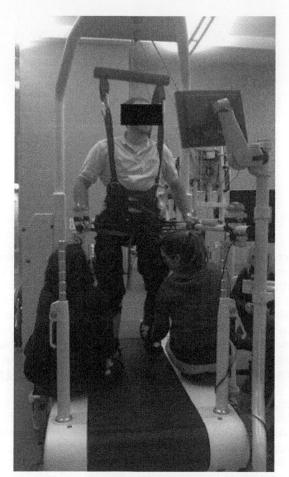

Fig. 2. Body weight–supported treadmill training (Andago with Woodway S55 treadmill (Hocoma AG, Switzerland)).

self-correct movement, which may be beneficial to ambulatory rehabilitation.[60] The contribution of therapist or robotic assistance to BWSTT may also be higher than other nontraditional training modalities, for instance, recumbent stepping, and may consequently result in less active contribution to training by the patient. Further, BWSTT involves specialized equipment that requires highly trained personnel to operate and is costly to initiate and maintain. BWSTT is rarely available in community settings, and when it is available, it is often at a high cost to the user.

ZeroG Overground Gait and Balance Training System

The ZeroG (Artech, LLC, Bioness Inc, Valencia, CA)[61] overground gait and balance training system is one of the most recently developed training and rehabilitation tools. This system uses a supportive harness with body weight off-loading, similar to that used with BWSTT, although the supportive harness is attached to a motorized trolley that moves along an overhead ceiling-mounted track (**Fig. 3**).[61] By mounting the harness to a ceiling track, patients have the opportunity to move over a variety of

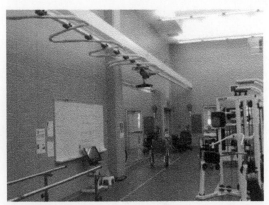

Fig. 3. ZeroG overhead track system (Artech, LLC, Bioness Inc, Valencia, CA).

surfaces and practice several different ambulatory movements (eg, forward and backward walking, turning, sitting-to-standing, balance activities). The ceiling-mounted track and supportive harness still allows for adjustment of the amount of body weight support provided, in the same manner as BWSTT, although it does not restrict patients to treadmill walking alone. The overhead motorized trolley system can be programmed to move with the patient or set to a stationary position.[61] Using this system, patients can participate safely in a variety of ambulatory or stationary movements, providing a natural progression from assisted treadmill training. The ZeroG training system also allows patients to practice ambulatory movements using their own assistive device.

The ZeroG overground gait and balance training system is a new tool to rehabilitation, and at this time there are no published data on its efficacy or clinical applicability. This system is extremely promising, however, considering the benefits of BWSTT in advanced neurologic disease populations and the additional applications of this training system. Specifically, the task-specific nature of this rehabilitation modality may translate into important improvements in walking and activities of daily living for adults with neurologic diseases. Although efficacy studies are clearly needed, this training modality will likely be appropriate for adults with a variety of neurologic diseases and disability levels because of the high level of customizability of this system.

The ZeroG training system is advantageous in that it is task specific and allows patients to practice walking and balance as well as specific tasks of daily living without the risk of falling. The variety of movements and actions possible with this training system also allows for a highly specialized and individualized training program.[61] This system would further be appropriate for patients with a variety of disability levels because of the supportive harness and body weight off-loading system. Similar to BWSTT, the most significant limitation is the high cost to purchase and maintain the system. The need for specialized facilities and personnel may also limit the widespread application of this rehabilitation modality.

TRADITIONAL VERSUS NONTRADITIONAL REHABILITATION STRATEGIES

The advantages and disadvantages of traditional and nontraditional rehabilitation modalities are summarized in **Table 1**. When comparing these rehabilitation strategies, a general tradeoff becomes evident; traditional modalities favor cost effectiveness and ease of implementation, whereas nontraditional modalities favor task specificity and

Table 1
Summary of advantages and disadvantages of traditional and nontraditional strategies for the rehabilitation of ambulatory limitations in adults with central neurologic disorders

Rehabilitation Modality	Advantages	Disadvantages
Traditional		
Exercise training	• Cost effective • Easy to implement • Can combine with other therapies	• Not task specific • Limited application for patients with high disability level
Conventional gait training	• Cost effective • Easy to implement • Task specific • Multitraining (ie, gait, balance, range of motion) • Individualized training • Can combine with other therapies	• Limited application for patients with high disability level • Requires specialized personnel (ie, physical or occupational therapists)
Nontraditional		
Functional electrical stimulation	• Can combine with other therapies	• Requires specialized equipment and personnel • Limited to individuals with intact lower motoneurons and peripheral nerves • Limited training time because of muscle fatigue • Peripheral nerve stimulation may cause pain
Recumbent stepper training	• Cost effective • Easy to implement • Applicable for all disability levels • Self-driven training system	• Movement restricted to stepping motion
Body weight–supported treadmill training	• Task specific • Applicable for all disability levels	• Movement restricted to treadmill walking • Costly to setup and maintain • Requires specialized personnel • Limited availability
ZeroG overground walking and balance system	• Task specific • Multitraining (ie, gait, balance, transfers) • Individualized training • Applicable for all disability levels	• Costly to setup and maintain • Requires specialized personnel • Limited availability

accessibility for those with severe mobility impairment. Some debate exists as to the advantage and potential benefit of nontraditional or advanced rehabilitation strategies and devices over traditional rehabilitation modalities. Considering the specialized and often costly nature of nontraditional rehabilitation, the efficacy of these modalities and the particular groups of patients for which they may be most appropriate should be established.

Few studies have compared traditional with nontraditional rehabilitation modalities using well-designed interventions. Two large randomized, controlled, multicenter trials have compared traditional rehabilitation with BWSTT in stroke[62] and SCI.[63] Duncan and colleagues[62] examined the effects of 36 sessions (90 minutes per session) of early therapist-assisted BWSTT (2 months after stroke), late therapist-assisted BWSTT (6 months after stroke), or home-based exercise (ie, flexibility, range of motion, upper and lower extremity strength, coordination, and static and dynamic balance training focus) in 408 patients. Similar improvements in ambulatory outcomes were observed regardless of the training intervention. Further, no differences in ambulatory outcomes were observed when patients were stratified by initial severity of walking impairment. A 12-week inpatient rehabilitation program compared conventional overground mobility therapy (ie, stretching, standing, and overground walking) with therapist-assisted BWSTT and overground walking practice in 146 patients with acute incomplete SCI.[63] Similar improvements in ambulatory outcomes were observed in both groups. These large-scale, well-designed interventions suggest similar efficacy of BWSTT and traditional rehabilitation strategies for improving ambulatory outcomes in patients with acute stroke and SCI. Other studies, however, have found superiority of BWSTT over traditional rehabilitation in patients with MS and PD.[54,64]

Importantly, for individuals with severe mobility impairment, most traditional rehabilitation strategies are not accessible. Nontraditional rehabilitation modalities may also be more effective for those with limited mobility. For instance, robot-assisted BWSTT with standard physiotherapy was compared with standard physiotherapy alone in inpatient subacute stroke rehabilitation.[65] Standard physiotherapy focused on movement of the paretic limb, upper-limb exercises, balance, standing, sitting, and transferring. BWSTT with standard physiotherapy was found to be more effective than standard physiotherapy alone on outcomes of mobility and function for individuals with severe motor impairment; however, there was no difference between treatments in those with less motor impairment. This finding suggests that the efficacy of nontraditional rehabilitation strategies may be dependent on the disability level of the patient. Similarly, improvements in balance and motor impairment were observed after recumbent stepper training but not a home-based exercise program involving movements of the affected lower limb in chronic stroke patients.[46] The cost-effective and accessible features of the recumbent stepper make it a particularly feasible tool for the rehabilitation of individuals with severe mobility impairments. Future trials should compare the effects of recumbent stepper training to BWSTT, as well as traditional rehabilitation, to determine the potential of this rehabilitation tool.

SUMMARY

The rehabilitation of ambulatory limitations in individuals with CNS disorders requires an individualized approach, with consideration to the specific deficits and rehabilitation targets for each individual. The level of neurologic impairment may be a primary determinant of the initial course of rehabilitation. The neurologic course of the disease itself, for instance stable (ie, chronic stroke) versus progressive (ie, MS), may also determine the course of rehabilitation strategies. Deficits that may contribute to ambulatory limitations such as muscle weakness, spasticity, fatigue, visuospatial deficits, cognitive impairment, and comorbid disease conditions should be evaluated and considered when selecting the most appropriate rehabilitation strategies. Social and environmental factors are also important considerations.

Traditional and nontraditional strategies should be considered complementary, rather than exclusive therapies, to provide the most effective ambulatory rehabilitation program. Different modalities can be used concomitantly or in succession, for example, a more intensive nontraditional intervention can be used initially (often in combination with traditional therapy) followed by traditional therapy alone (often in combination with exercise modalities performed independently by the patient), with final transition to home or community-based exercise. Further research is needed to better define the most appropriate strategies for specific patient groups (or specific levels of disability) and the outcomes of combined therapies.

REFERENCES

1. Minaire P. Disease, illness and health: theoretical models of the disablement process. Bull World Health Organ 1992;70:373–9.
2. Cameron MH, Wagner JM. Gait abnormalities in multiple sclerosis: pathogenesis, evaluation, and advances in treatment. Curr Neurol Neurosci Rep 2011;11(5): 507–15.
3. Pearson O, Busse M, van Deursen R, et al. Quantification of walking mobility in neurological disorders. QJM 2004;97(8):467–75.
4. Dickstein R. Rehabilitation of gait speed after stroke: a critical review of intervention approaches. Neurorehabil Neural Repair 2008;22(6):649–60.
5. Michael KM, Allen JK, Macko RF. Reduced ambulatory activity after stroke: the role of balance, gait, and cardiovascular fitness. Arch Phys Med Rehabil 2005; 86(8):1552–6.
6. Bloem BR, Hausdorff JM, Visser JE, et al. Falls and freezing of gait in Parkinson's disease: a review of two interconnected, episodic phenomena. Mov Disord 2004; 19(8):871–84.
7. Falvo MJ, Earhart GM. Six-minute walk distance in persons with Parkinson disease: a hierarchical regression model. Arch Phys Med Rehabil 2009;90(6):1004–8.
8. Allen NE, Sherrington C, Canning CG, et al. Reduced muscle power is associated with slower walking velocity and falls in people with Parkinson's disease. Parkinsonism Relat Disord 2010;16(4):261–4.
9. Allen NE, Sherrington C, Suriyarachchi GD, et al. Exercise and motor training in people with Parkinson's disease: a systematic review of participant characteristics, intervention delivery, retention rates, adherence, and adverse events in clinical trials. Parkinsons Dis 2012;2012:854328.
10. Stoller O, de Bruin ED, Knols RH, et al. Effects of cardiovascular exercise early after stroke: systematic review and meta-analysis. BMC Neurol 2012;12(1):45.
11. Hicks AL, Martin Ginis KA, Pelletier CA, et al. The effects of exercise training on physical capacity, strength, body composition and functional performance among adults with spinal cord injury: a systematic review. Spinal Cord 2011; 49(11):1103–27.
12. Dalgas U, Stenager E, Ingemann-Hansen T. Multiple sclerosis and physical exercise: recommendations for the application of resistance-, endurance- and combined training. Mult Scler 2008;14(1):35–53.
13. Brazzelli M, Saunders DH, Greig CA, et al. Physical fitness training for patients with stroke: updated review. Stroke 2012;43(4):e39–40.
14. Kjølhede T, Vissing K, Dalgas U. Multiple sclerosis and progressive resistance training: a systematic review. Mult Scler 2012. Available at: http://msj.sagepub.com/content/early/2012/04/24/1352458512437418. Accessed July 10, 2012.
15. David FJ, Rafferty MR, Robichaud JA, et al. Progressive resistance exercise and Parkinson's disease: a review of potential mechanisms. Parkinsons Dis 2012; 2012:124527.

16. Goodwin VA, Richards SH, Taylor RS, et al. The effectiveness of exercise interventions for people with Parkinson's disease: a systematic review and meta-analysis. Mov Disord 2008;23(5):631–40.
17. van de Port IG, Wood-Dauphinee S, Lindeman E, et al. Effects of exercise training programs on walking competency after stroke: a systematic review. Am J Phys Med Rehabil 2007;86(11):935–51.
18. Rampello A, Franceschini M, Piepoli M, et al. Effect of aerobic training on walking capacity and maximal exercise tolerance in patients with multiple sclerosis: a randomized crossover controlled study. Phys Ther 2007;87(5):545–59.
19. Dalgas U, Stenager E, Jakobsen J, et al. Resistance training improves muscle strength and functional capacity in multiple sclerosis. Neurology 2009;73(18): 1478–84.
20. Ferrante S, Ambrosini E, Ravelli P, et al. A biofeedback cycling training to improve locomotion: a case series study based on gait pattern classification of 153 chronic stroke patients. J Neuroeng Rehabil 2011;8:47.
21. Ambrosini E, Ferrante S, Pedrocchi A, et al. A novel biofeedback cycling training to improve gait symmetry in stroke patients: a case series study. IEEE Int Conf Rehabil Robot 2011;2011:5975495.
22. Ivey FM, Macko RF, Ryan AS, et al. Cardiovascular health and fitness after stroke. Top Stroke Rehabil 2005;12(1):1–16.
23. Haisma JA, van der Woude LH, Stam HJ, et al. Physical capacity in wheelchair-dependent persons with a spinal cord injury: a critical review of the literature. Spinal Cord 2006;44(11):642–52.
24. Koseoglu BF, Gokkaya NK, Ergun U, et al. Cardiopulmonary and metabolic functions, aerobic capacity, fatigue and quality of life in patients with multiple sclerosis. Acta Neurol Scand 2006;114(4):261–7.
25. Ng AV, Miller RG, Gelinas D, et al. Functional relationships of central and peripheral muscle alterations in multiple sclerosis. Muscle Nerve 2004;29(6):843–52.
26. Protas EJ, Stanley RK, Jankovic J, et al. Cardiovascular and metabolic responses to upper- and lower-extremity exercise in men with idiopathic Parkinson's disease. Phys Ther 1996;76(1):34–40.
27. Paul SS, Canning CG, Sherrington C, et al. Reduced muscle strength is the major determinant of reduced leg muscle power in Parkinson's disease. Parkinsonism Relat Disord 2012. Available at: http://www.ncbi.nlm.nih.gov/pubmed/22682756. Accessed June 9, 2012.
28. Warburton DE, Nicol CW, Bredin SS. Health benefits of physical activity: the evidence. CMAJ 2006;174(6):801–9.
29. Keus SH, Bloem BR, Hendriks EJ, et al. Evidence-based analysis of physical therapy in Parkinson's disease with recommendations for practice and research. Mov Disord 2007;22(4):451–60.
30. Alonso-Frech F, Sanahuja JJ, Rodriguez AM. Exercise and physical therapy in early management of Parkinson disease. Neurologist 2011;17:S47–53.
31. Salbach NM, Mayo NE, Wood-Dauphinee S, et al. A task-orientated intervention enhances walking distance and speed in the first year post stroke: a randomized controlled trial. Clin Rehabil 2004;18(5):509–19.
32. Zanca JM, Natale A, Labarbera J, et al. Group physical therapy during inpatient rehabilitation for acute spinal cord injury: findings from the SCIRehab Study. Phys Ther 2011;91(12):1877–91.
33. van Langeveld SA, Post MW, van Asbeck FW, et al. Contents of physical therapy, occupational therapy, and sports therapy sessions for patients with a spinal cord injury in three Dutch rehabilitation centres. Disabil Rehabil 2011;33(5):412–22.

34. Brown T, Kraft GH. Exercise and rehabilitation for individuals with multiple sclerosis. Phys Med Rehabil Clin N Am 2006;16:513–55.
35. Thaut MH, Abiru M. Rhythmic auditory stimulation in rehabilitation of movement disorders: a review of current research. Music Percept 2010;27(4):263–9.
36. Kadivar Z, Corcos DM, Foto J, et al. Effect of step training and rhythmic auditory stimulation on functional performance in Parkinson patients. Neurorehabil Neural Repair 2011;25(7):626–35.
37. Conklyn D, Stough D, Novak E, et al. A home-based walking program using rhythmic auditory stimulation improves gait performance in patients with multiple sclerosis: a pilot study. Neurorehabil Neural Repair 2010;24(9):835–42.
38. Thrasher TA, Popovic MR. Functional electrical stimulation of walking: function, exercise and rehabilitation. Ann Readapt Med Phys 2008;51(6):452–60.
39. Mushahwar VK, Jacobs PL, Normann RA, et al. New functional electrical stimulation approaches to standing and walking. J Neural Eng 2007;4(3):S181–97.
40. Sabut SK, Sikdar C, Kumar R, et al. Improvement of gait & muscle strength with functional electrical stimulation in sub-acute & chronic stroke patients. Conf Proc IEEE Eng Med Biol Soc 2011;2011:2085–8.
41. Liberson WT, Holmquest HJ, Scot D, et al. Functional electrotherapy: stimulation of the peroneal nerve synchronized with the swing phase of the gait of hemiplegic patients. Arch Phys Med Rehabil 1961;42:101–5.
42. Kottink AIR, Oostendorp LJM, Buurke JH, et al. The orthotic effect of functional electrical stimulation on the improvement of walking in stroke patients with a dropped foot: a systematic review. Artif Organs 2004;28(6):577–86.
43. Belda-Lois JM, Mena-del Horno S, Bermejo-Bosch I, et al. Rehabilitation of gait after stroke: a review towards a top-down approach. J Neuroeng Rehabil 2011; 8:66.
44. Field-Fote EC. Combined use of body weight support, functional electric stimulation, and treadmill training to improve walking ability in individuals with chronic incomplete spinal cord injury. Arch Phys Med Rehabil 2001;82(6):818–24.
45. Field-Fote EC, Roach KE. Influence of a locomotor training approach on walking speed and distance in people with chronic spinal cord injury: a randomized clinical trial. Phys Ther 2011;91(1):48–60.
46. Page SJ, Levine P, Teepen J, et al. Resistance-based, reciprocal upper and lower limb locomotor training in chronic stroke: a randomized, controlled crossover study. Clin Rehabil 2008;22(7):610–7.
47. Sage MD, Almeida QJ. Symptom and gait changes after sensory attention focused exercise vs aerobic training in Parkinson's disease. Mov Disord 2009; 24(8):1132–8.
48. Hass CJ, Garzarella L, de Hoyos DV, et al. Concurrent improvements in cardiorespiratory and muscle fitness in response to total body recumbent stepping in humans. Eur J Appl Physiol 2001;85(1–2):157–63.
49. Stoloff RH, Zehr EP, Ferris DP. Recumbent stepping has similar but simpler neural control compared to walking. Exp Brain Res 2007;178(4):427–38.
50. Moseley AM, Stark A, Cameron ID, et al. Treadmill training and body weight support for walking after stroke. Cochrane Database Syst Rev 2005;(4):CD002840.
51. Wessels M, Lucas C, Eriks I, et al. Body weight-supported gait training for restoration of walking in people with an incomplete spinal cord injury: a systematic review. J Rehabil Med 2010;42(6):513–9.
52. Swinnen E, Duerinck S, Baeyens JP, et al. Effectiveness of robot-assisted gait training in persons with spinal cord injury: a systematic review. J Rehabil Med 2010;42(6):520–6.

53. Swinnen E, Beckwée D, Pinte D, et al. Treadmill training in multiple sclerosis: can body weight support or robot assistance provide added value? A systematic review. Mult Scler Int 2012;2012:240274.

54. Picelli A, Melotti C, Origano F, et al. Robot-assisted gait training in patients with Parkinson disease: a randomized controlled trial. Neurorehabil Neural Repair 2012;26(4):353–61.

55. Picelli A, Melotti C, Origano F, et al. Does robotic gait training improve balance in Parkinson's disease? A randomized controlled trial. Parkinsonism Relat Disord 2012. Available at: http://www.ncbi.nlm.nih.gov/pubmed/22673035. Accessed June 12, 2012.

56. Hesse S, Schmidt H, Werner C, et al. Upper and lower extremity robotic devices for rehabilitation and for studying motor control. Curr Opin Neurol 2003;16(6): 705–10.

57. Lo AC, Triche EW. Improving gait in multiple sclerosis using robot-assisted, body weight supported treadmill training. Neurorehabil Neural Repair 2008;22(6): 661–71.

58. Westlake KP, Patten C. Pilot study of Lokomat versus manual-assisted treadmill training for locomotor recovery post-stroke. J Neuroeng Rehabil 2009;6:18.

59. Alcobendas-Maestro M, Esclarín-Ruz A, Casado-López RM, et al. Lokomat robotic-assisted versus overground training within 3 to 6 months of incomplete spinal cord lesion: Randomized controlled trial. Neurorehabil Neural Repair 2012. Available at: http://www.ncbi.nlm.nih.gov/pubmed/22699827. Accessed June 13, 2012.

60. Dobkin BH, Duncan PW. Should body weight-supported treadmill training and robotic-assistive steppers for locomotor training trot back to the starting gate? Neurorehabil Neural Repair 2012;26(4):308–17.

61. Available at: http://www.bioness.com/Healthcare_Professionals/Rehab_Center_Products/ZeroG.php. Accessed July 9, 2012.

62. Duncan PW, Sullivan KJ, Behrman AL, et al. Body-weight-supported treadmill rehabilitation after stroke. N Engl J Med 2011;364(21):2026–36.

63. Dobkin B, Apple D, Barbeau H, et al. Weight-supported treadmill vs over-ground training for walking after acute incomplete SCI. Neurology 2006;66(4):484–93.

64. Beer S, Aschbacher B, Manoglou D, et al. Robot-assisted gait training in multiple sclerosis: a pilot randomized trial. Mult Scler 2008;14(2):231–6.

65. Morone G, Bragoni M, Iosa M, et al. Who may benefit from robotic-assisted gait training? A randomized clinical trial in patients with subacute stroke. Neurorehabil Neural Repair 2011;25(7):636–44.

Assistive Devices for Ambulation

Joan E. Edelstein, MA, PT, FISPO, CPed

KEYWORDS

- Cane • Walker • Crutch • Walking • Assistive devices • Rehabilitation

KEY POINTS

- Assistive devices serve many functions to improve quality of life.
- Examination should include neuromuscular, cardiopulmonary, and orthopedic factors, as well as an assessment of the home environment and funding sources.
- Various designs are available.
- Fitting is critical to optimum function.
- Appropriate gait can maximize patient performance.

INTRODUCTION

For the patient with a central nervous system (CNS) disorder, assistive devices—canes, walkers, crutches, and orthoses—can make the difference between existing largely in the confines of home and engaging in the wider community. Ambulation aids have been used since the Neolithic period.[1,2]

Selecting the appropriate aid requires considering the amount of stability the patient requires for safe ambulation. For those with CNS disorders, device selection may progress from parallel bars to a large base quad cane and later to a single-point cane needed only when maneuvering outdoors, as neurologic recovery occurs, or in the reverse sequence, in the case of a progressive disorder.

Assistive devices serve one or more of the following functions:

- Improve balance
- Assist propulsion
- Reduce load on one lower limb or both
- Transmit sensory cues through the hands
- Obtain the physiologic benefits of upright posture
- Maneuver in places inaccessible to a wheelchair
- Notify passersby that the user requires special considerations, such as additional time when crossing streets or a taking a seat on the bus.

Technological advances in materials and designs have multiplied options. Changing demographics and social mores have broadened the market. No longer is it a rarity to

Program in Physical Therapy, College of Physicians and Surgeons, Columbia University, 710 West 18th Street, New York, NY 10032, USA
E-mail address: joaneedelstein@hotmail.com

Phys Med Rehabil Clin N Am 24 (2013) 291–303
http://dx.doi.org/10.1016/j.pmr.2012.11.001
1047-9651/13/$ – see front matter © 2013 Elsevier Inc. All rights reserved.

see someone in a shopping mall using a walker. Mobility-related assistive technology can be obtained through Medicare's durable medical equipment benefit[3] and the Department of Veterans Affairs.[4] Nevertheless, a nationwide sample of 3485 older Americans showed that income and insurance affect the use of canes and other assistive devices.[5]

The prescription should specify the aid most likely to maximize the patient's function; the individual's goals and personal preferences must be considered also. Ongoing device modification or progression from one aid to another is an additional responsibility of the clinician. Complexity and variability of funding sources add to the challenge of selecting the device that will meet a given patient's needs. Input from a physical therapist or an occupational therapist is often valuable in ensuring that the appropriate device is prescribed and in ensuring that the patient (and family, if appropriate) is trained adequately.

Key examination elements affecting device prescription are listed in **Table 1**. Even when deemed necessary and appropriately prescribed, some patients, when offered an assistive device, refuse, calling it a sign of disability or senility, or stating that they do not want to "give in" to their condition. It is therefore important that the clinician take the time to explain the rationale for using the device and its potential benefits.

CANES

Canes are the simplest aids for ambulation. They augment balance and provide sensory feedback from the walking surface. They are made from sturdy materials, such as walnut, oak, and other woods; metal, especially aluminum; and plastics, such as acrylics (eg, Lucite), fiberglass, and carbon fiber. Contemporary canes are sold in virtually every color of the rainbow and may display fanciful patterns.

Cane Designs

Unlike the walking stick, which usually is a straight shaft, perhaps topped by an ornamental knob, canes used in rehabilitation have a handle. Handles are often an inverted "U," which permits hanging the cane over the forearm or the back of a chair when not walking with it. A pistol grip handle and a shovel handle are other options. An ergonomically shaped handle (www.CanesCanada.com) is designed to contact more of the hand, thus contributing to the user's comfort; the handle is made for right and left hand use.

Table 1 Key elements of physical examination for assistive device prescription	
Neurologic factors	Coordination Balance Psychological, emotional, and cognitive state
Cardiopulmonary factors	Heart rate Blood pressure Aerobic capacity and endurance
Orthopedic factors	Flexibility and strength of hands, wrists, elbows, and shoulders Weight-bearing capacity of the lower limbs Availability of well-fitting shoes
Home environment	Space to ambulate Condition of walking surface Presence of stairs that may obstruct egress from the home
Funding	Insurance Personal financial resources

Cane shafts may be straight, offset, folding, or height-adjustable. Straight shafts are the least expensive and most durable. Folding canes are easier to store; an adult-size cane can be folded to approximately 30 cm.

The base of the cane usually is a single rubber tip, broad with deep grooves and kept clean to provide maximum traction. Other bases are standard and wide-based quadruped (quad), which features a distal rectangle supporting 4 tips, intended to increase the support area. Patients with hemiplegia may not find the 4-footed cane more advantageous than a single tip. Novel designs include the side walker/cane (www.tfihealthcare.com), which has 4 widely spaced rubber tips to increase stability, especially when used unilaterally by a patient with hemiplegia. Another base has a spring-loaded tip to absorb shock at initial contact. The Able Tripod (www.abletripodcane.com) has a flexible triangular tip which maintains floor contact at a wide range of shaft angles; this tip also absorbs shock and permits the cane to remain upright when not in use. A base with a retractable metal spike increases stability when the user walks on ice.

Cane Fitting

Whatever the device, it must fit properly so that the user can walk optimally. When being measured, the patient should wear the type of shoes that will be worn when using it. Elbows should be slightly flexed, about 30°. The tip of the cane is 5 to 10 cm lateral and 15 cm anterior to the shoe. The handle is approximately at the level of the ulnar styloid or greater trochanter. Canes with a broad base, rather than a single tip, should be positioned so that the edge that flares laterally faces away from the shoe. If the flared side is positioned medially, it might hit the ankle as the person enters the swing phase of gait.

Canes that are too long may skid, reducing support. Too short a cane imposes undue stress on the lumbosacral region. Shorter canes, however, enable healthy subjects to perceive ground touch more accurately than longer canes, suggesting that those with visual impairment will walk more safely with a slight decrease in cane length.[6-8]

Cane Gait

Most patients use a single cane held on the side opposite the affected (or more affected) leg. The user advances the cane and the affected foot and then steps forward with the unaffected foot. The cane augments balance via light support as well as provides sensory feedback from the walking surface. Haptic cues aid postural control in sighted and blind individuals, particularly when the cane is held in a slanted rather than a vertical position.[9]

The cane is usually kept on the floor during the stance phase on the paretic limb. A cane reduces force throughout the hip. Biomechanical modeling of cane use confirmed that it increases stability.[10] Blount's classic treatise, *Don't Throw Away the Cane*,[11] demonstrated how a cane reduces joint stress. Some individuals prefer to hold the cane in the ipsilateral hand, using the device to reduce foot contact force. A few people insist on using the cane in the dominant hand, regardless of the side of impairment.

Some people, especially those with balance difficulties, walk with a pair of canes.

Kinematic studies of patients with hemiparesis confirmed that a cane held on the uninvolved side reduced mediolateral and anteroposterior sway,[12] regardless of whether a standard or a 4-footed cane was used.[13-15] Subjects had longer stance time on the affected leg[16] and walked faster with a cane than without one.[17,18] Other research showed that cane use reduced erector spinae and tibialis anterior activity.[19] A cane is indicated for the patient who cannot apply at least 40% of their body weight to the paretic lower limb.[20] Post stroke patients who walked with a cane had poorer balance and less social participation than those who could manage unaided.[21] As compared with those who required a walker, however, cane users were less impaired.[22]

A cane is often the first assistive device used by patients with multiple sclerosis (MS) to increase walking velocity.[23] Other investigators confirm the utility of ambulatory aids, including canes, for patients with MS.[24–26]

A cane is often used by community-dwelling older adults to prevent falls.[27] A large-scale survey of older adults revealed that those in poorer health or who had more severe disability were more likely to use equipment rather than rely on personal assistance. A randomized controlled trial demonstrated that assistive technology reduced health care costs for older adults.[28]

WALKERS

Walkers are frames, usually aluminum, that provide bilateral support, eliminating the need to control a pair of canes or crutches.

Walker Designs

Walkers are available in many combinations:

- Base: 4 tips, 2 tips and 2 wheels, 4 wheels, 3 wheels
- Uprights: rigid, folding, reciprocating, stair climbing
- Proximal portion: hand grips, platform

The simplest model of walker has 4 legs, each ending in a rubber tip to improve traction. The 4-tip walker provides maximum stability, but must be lifted with each step. They are especially appropriate for high-friction surfaces, such as carpet and grass. Walkers with wheels can be pushed forward to provide moderate stability; they are easier to manage on smooth surfaces, such as hardwood flooring. Wheeled walkers, however, are relatively bulky, thus more difficult to stow in a car.

Other bases with 2 front wheels and 2 crutch tips are available. Two-wheeled walkers may have tennis balls or other glides on the rear uprights to smooth ambulation. The folding steel U-Step (www.ActiveForever.com) has a padded seat, hand brakes, and an optional laser light, intended to encourage patients with Parkinson disease to step forward. A walker can have a reciprocating mechanism to accommodate stairs, such as the Universal Stair Climbing Walker (www.tfihealthcare.com).

Uprights are vertical or angled and may be height-adjustable. Nova 4900 Traveler 3-wheeled walker (www.HealthyLegs.com) has 3 uprights each ending in a wheel. It is easier to maneuver in narrow corridors compared with a 4-wheeled walker. Wide-wheeled and four-tip walkers accommodate obese patients.

Handles may be rubberized grips or platforms. Direct-forming plastic can be used to make the handle more comfortable. The 4-legged hemi-walker with an arm platform is used on one side of the body, in place of a cane. The hemi-walker is more stable than the single-tipped cane.

Users can add a basket or fabric bag to their walkers. Some devices have a hinged seat with a compartment to hold small articles.

On-going governmental research is being conducted to develop a feasible robotic walker.[29]

Walker Fitting

A properly fitted walker allows the user's center of gravity to stay within the walker's base. Poor fitting could lead to loss of balance. The elbows should be flexed 15°, with the ulnar styloid at each walker's handle. Slight elbow flexion allows for downward push, allowing the patient to bear some weight through the upper limbs.[30,31]

If the handles are too low, the user risks keeping the elbows extended, eventually being drawn into excessive trunk forward flexion. Trunk flexion can inhibit hip extension during the stance phase of walking. The anterior position of the patient's center of gravity interferes with forward weight shifting, making it difficult to achieve adequate propulsion.

Unduly high handles may oblige the patient to flex the elbows too much and lean excessively onto the walker. The patient who compensates by pushing the walker too far from the trunk risks falling if the person's center of gravity is behind the walker's base of support.

Walker Gait

The patient advances the walker so that all tips touch the floor simultaneously. Walkers with wheels should be pushed forward slightly. With either design, the user then steps forward with one foot, following with the other foot. Biomechanical analysis with healthy young adults indicated that hand loads vary with the type of walker gait.[32] Hip flexion angle determines weight-bearing force during walker gait.[33] Walker use reduced vastus lateralis and soleus electromyographic activity.[34] Heart rate and oxygen consumption are appreciably higher with a 4-tipped walker compared with a rolling walker.[35,36]

Among adults with stroke, walkers improved functional mobility.[37–39] People with Parkinson disease demonstrate slower gait when using a walker compared with unaided gait.[40,41] Those with Huntington disease performed better with a wheeled walker than with canes or a 4-tip walker.[42]

Elderly adults walked more slowly with a rolling walker than unaided[43] but did not lag in achieving functional gains in rehabilitation.[44]

Although walkers improve patient stability, they do not eliminate the risk of falling. Those who require walkers have greater physical limitations, resulting in increased fall risk.[45] Forward-leaning posture is common and is associated with falls.[46] An analysis of 47,312 older adult fall injuries confirmed that walkers were involved in 7 times as many injuries as canes.[47]

CRUTCHES

Four major types of crutches are as follows:

- Underarm
- Triceps
- Forearm (Lofstrand)
- Platform

Underarm crutches are usually made of wood, aluminum, and titanium. They are also known as axillary crutches because the top of the crutch is sometimes termed the axillary piece. The axilla should *never* be used as a support area because the crutch may impinge on superficial nerves and vessels. The top is often covered with sponge rubber to increase friction and cushion stress against the chest. One design has a longer top to provide more chest support.[48] Energy cost with this design is less during the first minutes of walking, but does not differ from the efficiency of ordinary crutches for longer durations. The Easy Strutter Functional Orthosis (www.orthoticmobility.com) has a crutch top that includes, in addition to the underarm piece, a cushioned strap over the shoulder to distribute weight broadly. When 3-point gait with axillary crutches was compared with performance with the Easy Strutter, the latter imposed less stress on the palms; subjects also reported feeling more secure on level surfaces and stairs with them.[49]

The shape of the crutch handle does not seem to affect function or comfort.[50] The handle should have a resilient cover to cushion palmar compression. Metal crutches have spring-loaded detents that facilitate adjustment of hand grip height and overall crutch length. Wooden crutches include wing nuts for handle placement.

The traditional shaft bifurcates partway up from the base; however, streamlined single shaft crutches are widely available. Many tips described for canes can also be used on crutches. The Safe Walk (www.sailmarket.com) has 2 shafts both ending with rubber tips; one tip is always on the ground regardless of the angle of the crutch. A spring-loaded mechanism at the distal end of the shaft absorbs considerable impact shock. Rocker bottom crutches have 2 shafts that terminate distally in a curved piece. Ambulation with these crutches may lower energy consumption.[51–53]

Triceps crutches are made of aluminum. They were developed at the Roosevelt Institute for Rehabilitation, Warm Springs, GA during the 20th century poliomyelitis epidemic. The crutch is intended for patients with paralyzed shoulder muscles. The proximal portion of each crutch has medial and lateral uprights joined by a pair of posterior bands that keep the elbow extended, mimicking the action of the triceps. The upper cuff should contact the proximal third of the upper arm, approximately 5 cm below the anterior axillary fold. The lower cuff should lie 1 to 4 cm below the olecranon, avoiding bony contact, yet providing adequate stability. The distal part of the crutch is a single shaft.

Forearm (Lofstrand) crutches are usually made of aluminum with a vinyl-covered steel forearm cuff. Length and cuff position are adjustable. One innovation is made of compliant plastic with an S-curved shaft to absorb shock.[54] A variation of the rigid cuff is a leather cuff, sometimes known as the Kenny Armband. It was named after Sister Kenny, a nurse who treated patients with poliomyelitis. The armband is less restrictive than the rigid cuff.

Platform crutches provide a trough to permit forearm weight-bearing for those who cannot tolerate weight transmission through the hand. The platform should be angled so that the forearm rests at a 90-degree angle to the upper arm, maximizing comfort and control of the crutch.

Crutch Fitting

The underarm crutch should extend from a point approximately 4 to 5 cm (2 fingerbreadths) below the axilla to a point on the floor 5 cm lateral and 15 cm anterior to the shoe. The hand piece should enable the elbow to flex 30°. Slightly less flexion is suitable for the person who uses the 2-, 3-, or 4-point gait. More flexion is required for gaits that require the user to raise both feet from the floor simultaneously, such as the drag-to, swing-to, and swing-through patterns.

Crutches that are too short compel the user to lean forward, whereas those that are too long force the shoulders up and risk compression of the radial nerve or suprascapular nerve. Even when crutches are adjusted properly, if used incorrectly, some patients experience redness, pain, and abrasion of the lateral chest; tenderness over the medial aspect of the arm; cramping of the triceps; bruising of the medial epicondyle; shoulder pain; and ulnar neuropathy.

Crutch Gaits

Crutches are ordinarily used in pairs. With a single crutch, gait kinematics are asymmetrical.

Selection of gait pattern depends on the patient's ability to move the feet recipro-cally, tolerate full load on each leg, lift the body off the floor by pressing on the hands, and maintain balance. A habitual gait pattern may be altered when the patient encoun-ters a crowded environment or a slipping or sloping floor.

- Alternating (reciprocal) gait pattern: most individuals move reciprocally, one foot at a time, alternating with the crutch. Alternating gaits are relatively stable and less stressful on the cardiovascular system and the upper limbs, but movement may be rather slow.
- Four-point gait: the patient advances the right crutch, then the left foot, then the left crutch, followed by the right foot. This gait is the most stable gait pattern.[55]
- Two-point gait: the patient advances the right crutch and the left foot simulta-neously, followed by the left crutch and the right foot.
- Three-point gait: the patient advances both crutches together with the affected foot, then advances the unaffected foot. The three-point gait reduces load on the affected leg.

Swinging (simultaneous) gait patterns require reducing or eliminating load from both feet by forceful bilateral shoulder depression and elbow extension.

- Drag-to gait: both crutches are advanced, either individually or together, followed by dragging both feet on the floor to an imaginary line just behind the crutches.
- Swing-to gait: both crutches are advanced individually or together, followed by swinging the feet slightly off the floor to a point just behind the crutches.
- Swing-through gait: both crutches are advanced together, followed by swinging the feet beyond the line of the crutches. The swing-through gait is the fastest mode of crutch ambulation but requires the most floor space. The patient must be able to support the trunk and lower limbs for a period of time long enough to allow the legs to swing from behind to a position in front of the crutches. In addition, the patient must have confident balance when the posteriorly placed crutches are out of sight.

Ambulating with assistive devices imposes physiologic stresses on the patient, as indicated by elevated heart rate and energy expenditure. Use is particularly high with the swing-through gait because of large muscular demands in the upper limbs to lift the trunk and legs to initiate the body-swing phase and then to provide stability while the patient swings beyond the line of the crutches. Lacking the normal shock-absorbing function of the lower limbs, the patient absorbs the shock of ground contact with the crutch tips and the upper limbs.[56–58]

Although more than 90% of patients with spinal cord injury use a wheelchair,[59] some with incomplete spinal cord injury are able to ambulate with assistive devices, toler-ating higher than normal shoulder force.[60] Crutches enable faster gait than a walker with less energy demand.[61,62]

ORTHOSES AND "ACTIVE" DEVICES

In addition to canes and crutches, many people with stroke, spinal cord injury, MS, and other CNS disorders benefit from orthoses, particularly ankle-foot (AFO) designs. The simplest design is the posterior leaf spring AFO. Made of plastic, carbon fiber, or other lightweight flexible materials, it has a foot plate that lies under the plantar surface of the foot. The plate is continuous with an upright that covers much of the posterior calf. The upright terminates in a band just below the fibular head. The posterior leaf spring AFO maintains the foot in a neutral position during the swing phase, preventing the wearer from dragging the toe and tripping. Hinged AFOs allow dorsiflexion movement, while still avoiding foot drop. An adjustable plantarflexion stop can be added to produce a few degrees of forced dorsiflexion during the stance phase, with the aim of limiting hyperextension of the knee. An AFO with an anterior shell, sometimes called "ground reaction AFO," is less frequently prescribed; it induces a knee extension moment at the beginning of stance phase.

Functional electrical stimulation (FES) is an alternative to an AFO for some people with upper motor neuron lesions, particularly stroke. Various commercial systems all have a leg cuff with a battery-operated electrical stimulator and an electrode worn over the peroneal nerve. In one device, an accelerometer determines when the affected leg is in swing phase; at that time, dorsiflexors are stimulated to prevent the forefoot from dragging. Other devices rely on a heel switch to trigger dorsiflexor stimulation. As compared with an AFO, FES resulted in moderate gait improvement.[63–65] FES is described in greater detail elsewhere in this issue.

Patients with spinal cord injury and other neurologic disorders resulting in paraplegia often require knee-ankle-foot orthoses in addition to crutches for standing and walking. The usual knee-ankle-foot orthoses consist of a foot plate, bilateral uprights, knee hinges, and calf and thigh cuffs. Although knee hinges usually have a locking mechanism to prevent knee flexion, some hinges are designed to move freely when the patient is in the swing phase and then provide stance stability when the individual bears weight.[66] Newer approaches for patients with paraplegia are electrically powered hip-knee-ankle-foot orthoses that move mechanical hip and knee joints[67] and robotic exoskeletons.[68]

A hip flexion assist device was designed to compensate for hip flexor weakness, which, in addition to foot drop, often decreases foot clearance in patients with CNS disorders. The hip flexion assist device consists of 2 tension belts on each side of the leg, attached proximally to a belt worn around the waist, and distally to the patient's shoe. A pilot study on 21 patients with MS showed improved performance on timed walking tests, and a slight improvement of hip flexor strength on the leg wearing the device, and raised no significant safety concerns.[69]

COMPLICATIONS OF AMBULATORY DEVICES

Although assistive devices can improve balance and mobility, they may impose intolerable strength and metabolic demands.[70] Musculoskeletal and neurovascular complications are not uncommon with improperly fitted or incorrectly used canes, walkers, and crutches. Injury to the radial,[71–73] ulnar,[74] median,[75] and suprascapular nerves[76] occasionally occurs. Some people develop painful abrasion of the lateral chest; shoulder pain; tenderness or bruising over the medial aspect of the arm; cramping of the triceps; wrist osteoarthritis and undue ulnar bone stress; or any combination of these disorders. Improperly fitted or used underarm crutches can cause axillary artery thrombosis.[77–80] Orthoses are generally safe, but immobilization of the limb segments may lead to muscle atrophy and increased weakness, and abnormal pressure points may cause pain and pressure ulcers if the orthosis is not properly fitted. One study found that AFOs have a negative impact on dynamic balance in patients with MS.[81]

SUMMARY

Interacting with other people and the environment is fundamental to quality of life. Canes, walkers, and crutches increase, maintain, or improve functional capabilities of many individuals with neurologic disorders. Canes, the simplest assistive device for mobility, offer a choice of handle, shaft, and base. Walkers have various types of base, uprights, hand grips, platforms, and accessories. Crutch designs include underarm, triceps, forearm, and platform. Fitting assistive devices properly can avoid nerve and vascular compression and other complications of misfit or misuse. Many patients with hemiplegia wear ankle-foot orthoses to prevent toe drag during the swing phase. Knee-ankle-foot and higher orthoses are often prescribed for patients with paraplegia to enable standing and walking, usually with crutches. Some orthoses include electronic mechanisms to facilitate ambulation.

REFERENCES

1. Epstein S. Art, history and the crutch. Ann Med Hist 1937;9:304.
2. Loebl WY, Nunn JF. Staffs as walking aids in ancient Egypt and Palestine. J R Soc Med 1997;90:450–4.
3. Wolff JL, Agree EM, Kasper JD. Wheelchairs, walkers, and canes: what does Medicare pay for, and who benefits? Health Aff 2005;24:1140–9.
4. Winkler SL, Vogel B, Hoenig H, et al. Cost, utilization, and policy of provision of assistive technology devices to veterans post stroke by Medicare and VA. Med Care 2010;48:558–62.
5. Mathieson KM, Kronenfeld JJ, Keith VM. Maintaining functional independence in elderly adults: the roles of health status and financial resources in predicting home modifications and use of mobility equipment. Gerontologist 2002;42:24–31.
6. Dean E, Ross J. Relationships among cane fitting, function, and falls. Phys Ther 1993;73:494–500.
7. Lu CL, Yu B, Basford JR, et al. Influences of cane length on the stability of stroke patients. J Rehabil Res Dev 1997;34:91–100.
8. Dean E, Ross J. Movement energetics of individuals with a history of poliomyelitis. Arch Phys Med Rehabil 1993;74:478–83.
9. Boonsinsukh R, Panichareon L, Saengsirisuwan V, et al. Clinical identification for the use of light touch cues with a cane in gait rehabilitation post stroke. Top Stroke Rehabil 2011;18(Suppl 1):633–42.
10. Tagawa Y, Shiba N, Matsuo S, et al. Analysis of human abnormal walking using a multi-body model: joint models for abnormal walking and walking aids to reduce compensatory action. J Biomech 2000;33:1405–14.
11. Blount WP. Don't throw away the cane. J Bone Joint Surg Am 1956;18:695–708.
12. Maeda A, Nakamura K, Higuchi S, et al. Postural sway during cane use by patients with stroke. Am J Phys Med Rehabil 2001;80:903–8.
13. Milczarek JJ, Kirby RL, Harrison ER, et al. Standard and four-footed canes, their effect on the standing balance of patients with hemiparesis. Arch Phys Med Rehabil 1993;74:281–5.
14. Laufer Y. Effects of one-point and four-point canes on balance and weight distribution in patients with hemiparesis. Clin Rehabil 2002;16:141–8.
15. Laufer Y. The effect of walking aids on balance and weight-bearing patterns on patients with hemiparesis in various stance positions. Phys Ther 2003;83:112–22.
16. Beauchamp MK, Skrela M, Southmayd D, et al. Immediate effects of cane use on gait symmetry in individuals with subacute stroke. Physiother Can 2009;61:154–609.
17. Chen CL, Chen HC, Wong MK, et al. Temporal stride and force analysis of cane-assisted gait in people with hemiplegic stroke. Arch Phys Med Rehabil 2001;82:43–8.
18. Polese JC, Teixeira-Salmela LF, Nascimento LR, et al. The effects of walking sticks on gait kinematics and kinetics with chronic stroke survivors. Clin Biomech (Bristol, Avon) 2012;27:131–7.

19. Buurke JH, Mermens JH, Erren-Wolters CV, et al. The effect of walking aids on muscle activation patterns during walking in stroke patients. Gait Posture 2005; 22:164–70.

20. Guillebastre B, Roughier PR, Sibille B, et al. When might a cane be necessary for walking following a stroke? Neurorehabil Neural Repair 2012;26:173–7.

21. Hamzat TK, Kobiri A. Effects of walking with a cane on balance and social participation among community-dwelling post-stroke individuals. Eur J Phys Rehabil Med 2008;44:121–6.

22. Jutai J, Coulson S, Teasell R, et al. Mobility assistive device utilization in a prospective study of patients with first-ever stroke. Arch Phys Med Rehabil 2007;88:1268–75.

23. Gianfrancesco MA, Triche EW, Fawcett JA, et al. Speed- and cane-related alterations in gait parameters in individuals with multiple sclerosis. Gait Posture 2011; 33:140–2.

24. Blake DJ, Bodine CJ. An overview of assistive technology for persons with multiple sclerosis. J Rehabil Res Dev 2002;39:299–312.

25. Fay BT, Boninger ML. The science behind mobility devices for individuals with multiple sclerosis. Med Eng Phys 2002;24:375–83.

26. Souza A, Kelleher A, Cooper R, et al. Multiple sclerosis and mobility-related assistive technology: systematic review of literature. J Rehabil Res Dev 2010;47: 213–23.

27. Aminzadeh F, Edwards N. Factors associated with cane use among community dwelling older adults. Public Health Nurs 2000;17:474–83.

28. Mann WC, Ottenbacher KJ, Fraas L, et al. Effectiveness of assistive technology and environmental interventions in maintaining independence and reducing home care costs for the frail elderly: a randomized controlled trial. Arch Fam Med 1999;8:210–7.

29. Rentschler AJ, Cooper RA, Blasch B, et al. Intelligent walkers for the elderly: performance and safety testing of VA-PAMAID robotic walker. J Rehabil Res Dev 2003;40:423–31.

30. Takanokura M. Optimal handgrip height of four-wheeled walker on various road conditions to reduce muscular load for elderly users with steady walking. J Biomech 2010;22:843–8.

31. Takanokura M. Theoretical optimization of usage and four-wheeled walker and body posture of elderly users for comfortable steady walking. Conf Proc IEEE Eng Med Biol Soc 2008;2008:4519–22.

32. Bachschmidt RA, Harris GF, Simoneau GG. Walker-assisted gait in rehabilitation: a study of biomechanics and instrumentation. IEEE Trans Neural Syst Rehabil Eng 2001;9:96–105.

33. Ishikura T. Biomechanical analysis of weight bearing force and muscle activation levels in the lower extremities during gait with a walker. Acta Med Okayama 2001; 55:73–82.

34. Clark BC, Manini TM, Ordway NR, et al. Leg muscle activity during walking with assistive devices at varying levels of weight bearing. Arch Phys Med Rehabil 2004;85:1555–60.

35. Cetin E, Muzembo J, Pardessus V, et al. Impact of different types of walking aids on the physiological energy cost during gait for elderly individuals with several pathologies and dependent on a technical aid for walking. Ann Phys Rehabil Med 2010;53:399–405.

36. Priebe JR, Kram R. Why is walker-assisted gait metabolically expensive? Gait Posture 2011;34:265–9.

37. Paquet N, Desrosiers J, Demers L, et al. Predictors of daily mobility skills 6 months post-discharge from acute care or rehabilitation in older adults with stroke living at home. Disabil Rehabil 2009;31:1267–74.
38. Tyson SF. The support taken through walking aids during hemiplegic gait. Clin Rehabil 1998;12:395–401.
39. Tyson SF, Rogerson L. Assistive walking devices in nonambulant patients undergoing rehabilitation. Arch Phys Med Rehabil 2009;90:475–9.
40. Cubo E, Moore CG, Leurgans S, et al. Wheeled and standard walkers in Parkinson's disease patients with gait freezing. Parkinsonism Relat Disord 2003;10:9–14.
41. Bryant MS, Pourmoghaddam A, Thrasher A. Gait changes in walking devices in persons with Parkinson's disease. Disabil Rehabil Assist Technol 2011;7:149–52.
42. Kloos AD, Kegelmeyer DA, White SE, et al. The impact of different types of assistive devices on gait measures and safety in Huntington's disease. PLoS One 2012;7:e30903.
43. Liu HH, McGee M, Wang W, et al. Comparison of gait characteristics between older rolling walker users and older potential walker users. Arch Gerontol Geriatr 2009;48:276–80.
44. Vogt L, Lucki K, Bach M, et al. Rollator use and functional outcomes of geriatric rehabilitation. J Rehabil Res Dev 2010;47:151–6.
45. Andersen DA, Roos BA, Stanziano DC, et al. Walker use, but not falls, is associated with lower physical functioning and health of residents in an assisted-living environment. Clin Interv Aging 2007;2:123–37.
46. Liu HH. Assessment of rolling walkers used by older adults in senior-living communities. Geriatr Gerontol Int 2009;9:124–30.
47. Stevens JA, Thomas K, The L, et al. Unintentional fall injuries associated with walkers and canes in older adults treated in U.S. emergency departments. J Am Geriatr Soc 2009;57:1464–9.
48. Hinton CA, Cullen KE. Energy expenditure during ambulation with Ortho crutches and axillary crutches. Phys Ther 1982;62:813–9.
49. Nyland J, Bernasek T, Markee B, et al. Comparison of the Easy Strutter Functional Orthosis System™ and axillary crutches during modified 3-point gait. J Rehabil Res Dev 2004;41:195–206.
50. Sala DA, Leva LM, Kummer FJ, et al. Crutch handle design: effect on palmar loads during ambulation. Arch Phys Med Rehabil 1998;79:1473–6.
51. Basford JR, Rhetta HL, Schleusner MP. Clinical evaluation of the rocker bottom crutch. Orthopedics 1990;13:457–60.
52. Nielsen DH, Harris JM, Minton YM, et al. Energy cost, exercise intensity, and gait efficiency of standard versus rocker-bottom axillary crutch walking. Phys Ther 1990;70:487–93.
53. Requejo PS, Wahl DP, Bontrager EL, et al. Upper extremity kinetics during Lofstrand crutch-assisted gait. Med Eng Phys 2005;27:19–29.
54. Shortell D, Kucer J, Neeley WL, et al. The design of a compliant composite crutch. J Rehabil Res Dev 2001;38:23–32.
55. Babic J, Karcnik T, Bajd T. Stability analysis of four-point walking. Gait Posture 2001;14:56–60.
56. Thys H, Willems PA, Snels P. Energy cost, mechanical work and muscular efficiency in swing-through gait with elbow crutches. J Biomech 1996;29:1473–82.
57. Noreau L, Richards CL, Comeau F, et al. Biomechanical analysis of swing-through gait in paraplegic and non-disabled individuals. J Biomech 1995;28:689–700.

58. Rovic JS, Childress DS. Pendular model of paraplegic swing-through crutch ambulation. J Rehabil Res Dev 1988;25:1–16.
59. Biering-Sorensen F, Hansen RB, Biering-Sorensen J. Mobility aids and transport possibilities 10-45 years after spinal cord injury. Spinal Cord 2004;42:699–706.
60. Haubert LL, Gutierrez DD, Newsam CJ, et al. A comparison of shoulder joint forces during ambulation with crutches versus a walker in persons with incomplete spinal cord injury. Arch Phys Med Rehabil 2006;87:63–70.
61. Melis EH, Torres-Moreno R, Barbeau H, et al. Analysis of assisted-gait characteristics in persons with incomplete spinal cord injury. Spinal Cord 1999;37:430–9.
62. Ulkar B, Yavuzer G, Buner R, et al. Energy expenditure of the paraplegic gait: comparison between different walking aids and normal subjects. Int J Rehabil Res 2003;26:213–7.
63. Bulley C, Shiels J, Wilkie K, et al. User experiences, preferences and choices relating to functional electrical stimulation and ankle foot orthoses for foot-drop after stroke. Physiotherapy 2011;97:226–33.
64. Israel S, Kotowski S, Talbott N, et al. The therapeutic effect of outpatient use of a peroneal nerve functional electrical stimulation neuroprosthesis in people with stroke: a case series. Top Stroke Rehabil 2011;18:738–45.
65. Ring H, Treger I, Gruendlinger L, et al. Neuroprosthesis for foot drop compared with an ankle-foot orthosis: effects on postural control during walking. J Stroke Cerebrovasc Dis 2009;18:41–7.
66. Davis PC, Bach TM, Pereira DM. The effect of stance control orthoses on gait characteristics and energy expenditure in knee-ankle-foot orthosis users. Prosthet Orthot Int 2010;34:206–15.
67. Farris RJ, Quintero HA, Goldfarb M. Preliminary evaluation of a powered low limb orthosis to aid walking in paraplegic individuals. IEEE Trans Neural Syst Rehabil Eng 2011;19:652–9.
68. Del-Ama AJ, Koutsou AD, Moreno JC, et al. Review of hybrid exoskeletons to restore gait following spinal cord injury. J Rehabil Res Dev 2012;49:497–514.
69. Sutliff M, Naft J, Stough D, et al. Efficacy and safety of a hip flexion assist orthosis in ambulatory multiple sclerosis patients. Arch Phys Med Rehabil 2008;89:1611–7.
70. Bateni H, Maki BE. Assistive devices for balance and mobility: benefits, demands, and adverse consequences. Arch Phys Med Rehabil 2005;86:134–45.
71. Rudin LN, Levine L. Bilateral compression of radial nerve (crutch paralysis). Phys Ther Rev 1951;31:229.
72. Ball NA, Stempien LM, Pasupuleti DV, et al. Radial nerve palsy: a complication of walker usage. Arch Phys Med Rehabil 1989;70:236.
73. Hug U, Burg D, Baldi SV, et al. Compression neuropathy of the radial palmar thumb nerve. Chir Main 2004;23:49–51.
74. Veerendrakumar M, Taly AB, Nagaraja D. Ulnar nerve palsy due to axillary crutch. Neurol India 2001;49:67–70.
75. Kellner WS, Felsenthal G, Anderson JM, et al. Carpal tunnel syndrome in the non-paretic hands of hemiplegics: stress-induced by ambulatory assistive devices. Orthop Rev 1986;15:608–11.
76. Shabes D, Scheiber M. Suprascapular neuropathy related to the use of crutches. Am J Phys Med 1986;65:298–9.
77. Platt H. Occlusion of the axillary artery due to pressure by a crutch. Arch Surg 1930;20:314–6.
78. Brooks AL, Fowler SB. Axillary artery thrombosis after prolonged use of crutches. J Bone Joint Surg Am 1964;46:863–4.

79. Feldman DR, Vujic I, McKay D, et al. Crutch-induced axillary artery injury. Cardiovasc Intervent Radiol 1995;18:296–9.
80. McFall B, Arya N, Soong C, et al. Crutch induced axillary artery injury. Ulster Med J 2004;73:50–2.
81. Cattaneo D, Marazzini F, Crippa A, et al. Do static or dynamic AFOs improve balance? Clin Rehabil 2002;16(8):894–9.

Technological Advances in Interventions to Enhance Poststroke Gait

Lynne R. Sheffler, MD[a],*, John Chae, MD[a,b]

KEYWORDS

- Gait • Hemiparesis • Motor relearning • Neuroplasticity

KEY POINTS

- Poststroke gait training interventions may be either therapeutic, resulting in enhanced motor recovery, or compensatory, whereby assistance or substitution for neurologic deficits results in improved functional performance.
- Functional electrical stimulation, body weight–supported treadmill training, and robotic-assisted gait training are examples of poststroke gait training therapies.
- Poststroke gait training therapies are predicated on activity-dependent neuroplasticity, which is the concept that cortical reorganization following central nervous system injury may be induced by repetitive, skilled, and cognitively engaging active movement.
- Additional research is necessary to determine whether specific technology-enhanced gait training methods are superior to conventional gait training methods.

INTRODUCTION

This article provides a comprehensive review of specific rehabilitation interventions used to enhance hemiparetic gait following stroke. Neurologic rehabilitation interventions may be considered either therapeutic or compensatory. Poststroke therapeutic interventions may improve gait performance by various motor relearning mechanisms including improved motor strength or enhanced motor control. Motor relearning is defined as the recovery of previously learned motor skills that have been lost following localized damage to the central nervous system.[1] Compensatory interventions may improve gait performance by providing assistance or by substituting for neurologic

This work was supported in part by grant K23HD060689 from the National Institute for Child Health and Human Development.

[a] Department of Physical Medicine and Rehabilitation, MetroHealth Medical Center, Cleveland Functional Electrical Stimulation Center, Case Western Reserve University, 2500 MetroHealth Drive, Cleveland, OH 44109, USA; [b] Department of Biomedical Engineering, Case Western Reserve University, 10900 Euclid Avenue, Cleveland, OH 44106, USA
* Corresponding author.
E-mail address: lsheffler@metrohealth.org

Phys Med Rehabil Clin N Am 24 (2013) 305–323
http://dx.doi.org/10.1016/j.pmr.2012.11.005

deficits to improve function. The specific spatiotemporal, kinematic, and kinetic parameters of gait that distinguish hemiparetic gait from other upper motor neuron gait patterns are described elsewhere in this issue. Included in this article are specific clinical and research applications of rehabilitation interventions that may enhance poststroke gait, including lower extremity functional electrical stimulation (FES), body weight–supported treadmill training (BWSTT), and lower extremity robotic-assisted gait training. These 3 poststroke gait training therapies are all predicated on activity-dependent neuroplasticity, which is the concept that cortical reorganization following central nervous system injury may be induced by repetitive, skilled, and cognitively engaging active movement. This article does not cover spasticity management, lower extremity orthotics, or specific physical therapy (PT) therapeutic treatments such as neurodevelopmental technique (NDT). Instead, this article provides a concise overview of evidence-based research that supports the efficacy of the 3 interventions mentioned earlier, as well as providing perspective on future developments to enhance poststroke gait in neurologic rehabilitation.

FUNCTIONAL ELECTRICAL STIMULATION FOR GAIT TRAINING

Neuromuscular electrical stimulation (NMES) refers to the activation of paretic or paralyzed muscles via stimulation of an intact lower motor neuron (LMN). The term FES was originally coined by Moe and Post[2] to describe the use of NMES to activate paretic muscles in a magnitude and sequence that directly facilitates a functional task such as walking. A lower extremity neuroprosthesis is an FES device or system designed to enhance functional walking, and the term neuroprosthetic effect describes the enhancement of walking performance that results when the neuroprosthesis is used. This effect may be evident by improved gait efficiency (for example, energy expenditure) or by improved spatiotemporal, kinematic, or kinetic parameters of gait (for example, walking velocity, paretic ankle dorsiflexion angle at heelstrike, or paretic plantarflexion power at push-off). Evolving basic science and clinical studies on central motor neuroplasticity support the role of active repetitive movement training of a paretic limb to enhance motor relearning, and thus lower extremity FES applications have also been proposed for therapeutic purposes in hemiparesis. The rationale for a therapeutic role of FES is that, if active repetitive movement training facilitates motor recovery, then, theoretically, FES-mediated repetitive movement training may also facilitate poststroke motor recovery. A recent review of the clinical and research applications of NMES in neurorehabilitation includes an overview of FES neurophysiology, FES componentry, and therapeutic applications of research and commercially available FES devices.[3]

Neurophysiology of FES

Most clinical FES applications are limited to patients with upper motor neuron dysfunction, because FES depends on the LMN being intact. Either the motor point of the nerve proximal to the neuromuscular junction or the peripheral nerve itself can be directly stimulated by clinical and research-based FES systems. The threshold for eliciting a nerve fiber action potential is 100 to 1000 times less than the threshold for muscle fiber stimulation.[4] An action potential (AP) induced by an FES system is identical to the all-or-none phenomenon of the AP produced by natural physiologic means. However, an AP produced by normal physiologic mechanisms initially recruits the smallest diameter neurons before recruitment of larger diameter fibers, such as α motor neurons.[5] The nerve fiber recruitment pattern induced by FES differs from a physiologic AP by following the principle of reverse recruitment order. Reverse recruitment order means that the nerve stimulus threshold is inversely proportional to the diameter of the neuron. Thus, large-diameter nerve fibers, which innervate large motor units, are recruited preferentially. Adjustment of stimulus parameters such as stimulus amplitude, pulse width, and frequency[4,6,7] thus affect both nerve fiber recruitment and resultant muscle contraction force characteristics. The minimum stimulus frequency that can generate a fused muscle response is approximately 12.5 Hz. Although stimulation frequencies higher than 12.5 Hz can generate higher muscle forces, there is a risk of muscle fiber fatigue and resultant decrease in muscle contractile force. An efficient FES system is designed to use the minimum stimulus frequency that produces a fused response,[8–10] with ideal stimulation frequencies ranging from 18 to 25 Hz for lower limb applications.

Components of FES Systems

Most research and commercially available FES systems for neurorehabilitation are in 2 broad categories based on electrode type: transcutaneous (surface) electrode and implanted electrode systems. A transcutaneous electrode is applied directly to the skin and stimulates either the peripheral nerve or the motor point of the underlying muscle. A transcutaneous electrode is the simplest electrode available and uses an external lead to connect directly to the neurostimulator device. An electrical current is created when 2 electrodes are placed in either a monopolar or bipolar configuration in relation to each other. The risk of tissue injury in patients with cognitive and/or sensory deficits may be increased with a transcutaneous electrode system and thus specific neurologic deficits must be evaluated before use. Other common limitations associated with transcutaneous electrode systems in patients who have had strokes include intolerance caused by activation of cutaneous pain receptors, poor muscle selectivity, inconsistency with electrode positioning, insecure fixation on a moving limb, skin irritation associated with the electrode, and cosmetic concerns.[3]

The percutaneous intramuscular electrode[11] is a type of implantable electrode. The placement of a percutaneous electrode is a minimally invasive procedure; however, lead wires that exit the skin are required to connect the electrode to the neurostimulator. The advantages and disadvantages of the percutaneous electrode have been well described previously.[3] The advantages of the percutaneous electrode are the elimination of skin resistance and cutaneous pain issues, greater muscle selectivity, and lower stimulation currents. Safety risks include lead displacement or breakage, infection, and granuloma formation associated with retained electrode fragments. The cumulative long-term failure rate of percutaneous electrodes varies between 56% and 80%,[12–14] which generally limits their use to less than 3 months. As a result, the most common applications of percutaneous electrodes are for time-limited therapeutic purposes or research applications.

Epimysial,[15–18] epineural, intraneural,[19–21] and cuff[22–25] electrodes are all types of surgically implanted electrodes that may be used for long-term neurostimulation applications. These electrodes are surgically placed above the muscle, above the nerve, within the nerve, or around the nerve, respectively. These types of implanted electrodes all connect to implanted lead wires and require the implantation of the neurostimulator. A radiofrequency (RF) telemetry link relays both power and command instructions to the neurostimulator from an external control unit. An implanted peroneal nerve stimulation (PNS) device[26–28] is an example of a clinically viable neuroprosthesis that uses implantable electrodes.

Correlating user intent to functional performance, particularly in the application of a lower extremity neuroprosthesis, presents significant challenges in the design of

FES control systems. Many upper extremity clinical FES systems use open-loop control (preset pattern of stimulation) with sensory feedback limited to residual visual and proprioceptive input. A closed-loop control system for continuous real-time modification of the stimulation pattern based on sensory feedback offers maximal advantage for a lower extremity neuroprosthesis. A transcutaneous PNS device is an example of a neuroprosthesis that uses a closed-loop control system such as a simple heel switch,[29] tilt sensor,[30] or acceleration sensor.[31]

Lower Extremity FES in Hemiparesis

The initial application of a neuroprosthesis in hemiparesis was the transcutaneous PNS device for correction of ankle dorsiflexion weakness associated with upper motor neuron dysfunction. In a 1961 publication, Lieberson[32] first described a stimulator that dorsiflexed the ankle during the swing phase of gait. Burridge and colleagues[29] later reported that chronic stroke survivors treated with PNS and PT had a significant increase in walking velocity and decrease in energy expenditure measured by the physiologic cost index compared with a control group who received PT only. The application of surface PNS has more recently been proposed as an alternative to an ankle-foot orthosis (AFO) based on other favorable neuroprosthetic effects of PNS.[33–35] Studies of hemiparetic subjects treated with neuroprosthetic applications of PNS have also reported possible therapeutic effects including enhanced walking speed,[34,36–38] increased maximal isometric contraction of the ankle dorsiflexors and plantarflexors,[39] increased dorsiflexion torque,[40] increased agonist electromyogram (EMG) activity and decreased EMG cocontraction ratios,[41] increased maximum root mean square (measure of muscle output capacity),[38] decreased calf spasticity,[38] and improved ankle control,[42] outcomes that were all measured while the subject was not wearing the device. Studies that have specifically compared the neuroprosthetic effect of a PNS with the orthotic effect of an AFO in hemiplegic gait[29,36,37,43,44] have also facilitated broader clinical prescription and usage of these devices.

The US Food and Drug Administration (FDA) has approved 3 surface PNS devices for clinical use in the United States. These devices are the Odstock Dropped Foot Stimulator (ODFS; Odstock Medical Limited, Salisbury, UK; **Fig. 1**), Ness L300 Footdrop System (Bioness Inc, Valencia, CA; **Fig. 2**), and the WalkAide System (Innovative Neurotronics, Austin, TX; **Fig. 3**).

The ODFS also carries the CE mark of approval by the European Union. The ODFS and the Ness L300 device use heel switches and the WalkAide device uses a tilt sensor as a control system to time stimulation to the swing phase of gait. The clinical use of these devices may be limited in patients who have had strokes who have skin breakdown or edema, lower extremity sensory deficits, cognitive deficits, ankle range-of-motion limitations, plantarflexion spasticity, cerebellar ataxia, and/or muscle fatigue. Common reasons for lack of efficacy of a surface PNS device include patient intolerance to surface stimulation, difficulty with electrode placement, insufficient medial-lateral control during stance phase, persistent genu recurvatum, and/or lack of rehabilitation support staff to assist with device programming.

The technical limitations of transcutaneous devices may ultimately be solved with the further refinement of implantable neurostimulation systems. Early studies first reported improvements in spatiotemporal gait parameters following implantation of a single-channel PNS device.[45,46] Although an implantable PNS device is not presently FDA approved in the United States, multichannel implantable PNS devices have recently undergone clinical investigation in Europe. A dual-channel device developed at the University of Twente and Roessingh Research and Development (The Netherlands) stimulates the deep and superficial peroneal nerves for better control

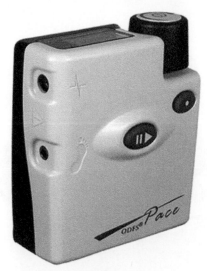

Fig. 1. The ODFS. (*Courtesy of* Odstock Medical Limited, The National Clinical FES Centre, Salisbury, UK; with permission.)

and balance of ankle dorsiflexion, eversion, and inversion.[47] A 4-channel device, developed at Aalborg University (Denmark) uses a nerve cuff electrode with 4 tripolar electrodes, oriented to activate different nerve fibers within the common peroneal nerve.[48] Both devices have received the CE mark approval in the European Union and clinical experience with these devices is now being reported. Recent clinical trials that have evaluated the efficacy of an implantable PNS device report a neuroprosthetic effect on walking speed,[27] paretic double support and nonparetic single support,[28] and ankle dorsiflexion angle during swing.[28] No PNS therapeutic effect was found in a study that compared 6 months of ambulation using an implantable, 2-channel peroneal nerve stimulator with an AFO[26]; however, increased voluntary muscle output of the tibialis anterior and gastrocnemius/soleus muscles in the PNS group were hypothesized to be evidence of neuroplasticity.

Several multichannel transcutaneous stimulation systems have been trialed that incorporate knee and hip flexion and extension as well as ankle dorsiflexion.[49–51] The rationale for these more complex stimulation systems is that poststroke gait

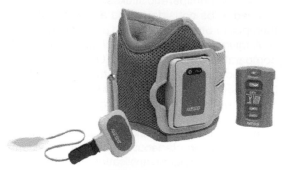

Fig. 2. The Bioness L300 Footdrop System. (*Courtesy of* Bioness Inc, Valencia, CA; with permission.)

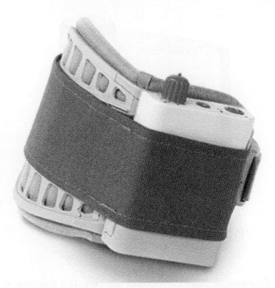

Fig. 3. The WalkAide System. (*Courtesy of* Innovative Neurotronics, Austin, TX; with permission.)

deviation associated with hemiplegia is not limited to ankle dysfunction or remedied by correction of footdrop alone. However, lower limb transcutaneous systems are particularly limited by reduced muscle selectivity, poor consistency of stimulation, and discomfort associated with sensory stimulation of larger, weight-bearing lower extremity muscles. From a clinical standpoint, as the number of electrodes increases, transcutaneous systems are increasingly difficult to clinically implement.[3] However, commercially available PNS devices including the Ness L300 Plus System and the Odstock 2 Channel Stimulator device have recent modifications that allow activation of additional muscles groups such as the quadriceps and/or hamstring muscles. Multichannel percutaneous lower limb systems[52,53] remain limited to research applications or time-limited therapeutic interventions intended to facilitate motor relearning as opposed to providing a longer-term neuroprosthetic solution.

Summary

A transcutaneous PNS device may be an appropriate clinical alternative to an AFO in select patients who have had hemiparetic strokes. Neurologic and medical issues that affect patient safety need to be considered and a device trial under the guidance of a trained physical therapist or other rehabilitation professional is recommended before device prescription. Additional practical issues, including access to long-term technical support and comparative device (PNS vs AFO) costs should also be considered. Additional research is necessary to determine the clinical efficacy of a 2-channel transcutaneous PNS device that incorporates quadriceps and/or hamstring stimulation. Clinical experience outside the United States suggests that an implantable PNS device may be a viable neuroprosthesis for select patients. However, potential benefits must be tempered with the risks and costs associated with an invasive procedure. At present, multichannel percutaneous lower limb FES systems remain limited to research and/or time-limited therapeutic applications. In addition, research is increasingly focusing on new technologies, such as harnessing cortical control signals, that may provide an enhanced means of interfacing with a neuroprosthesis,[54,55] and developing multichannel networked implantable neuroprostheses systems[56] that may someday address both upper and lower limb paralysis associated with central nervous system injury.

BODY WEIGHT-SUPPORTED TREADMILL TRAINING FOR GAIT TRAINING

BWSTT is an adaptive therapeutic training modality that allows otherwise nonambulatory or limited ambulatory patients who have had hemiparetic strokes to participate in task-specific gait training. Patients are fitted with harnesses that provide partial support of their full body weight as they are suspended over the treadmill surface. With the assistance of 1 or several physical therapists to facilitate paretic lower limb placement, balance, and limb sequencing, the patient is able to participate in repetitive gait training exercises while upright and partially weight bearing. The primary advantage of any BWSTT method is that the patient is able to safely be upright with limited physical assistance, which allows the treating physical therapist to observe and correct the gait pattern to improve functional performance.[57] Overground walking with partial body weight support (BWS), without the use of a treadmill, has been shown to improve walking in patients who have had hemiparetic strokes.[58,59] In a recent study, self-selected walking speeds over a 15-m walkway increased 17% on average when hemiparetic subjects walked with some level of BWS compared with the no-BWS condition.[59] Oxygen consumption (as measured by maximal oxygen uptake [Vo_2]) and heart rate were improved at both self-selected and maximum walking speeds during walking with 30% BWS on a treadmill compared with unsupported treadmill walking.[60] Hesse and colleagues[61] evaluated the gait patterns of hemiparetic subjects walking on a treadmill with 0%, 15%, and 30% BWS compared with overground walking. BWSTT was associated with a more prolonged single-stance period of the paretic limb, greater gait symmetry, less plantar flexor spasticity, and a more regular activation pattern of the gastrocnemius/soleus and anterior tibialis muscles compared with floor walking. Compared with overground walking or overground training using partial BWS, BWSTT may allow the therapist to achieve a more symmetric, efficient hemiparetic gait pattern within a more practical physical space.

Clinical Application of BWSTT Gait Training

Commercially available body weight–supported devices may have both overground and treadmill capability for use in a therapy gym or home setting. Examples of such devices include the body-weight support mechanism of the Lokomat System (Levi BWS, Hocoma, Zurich, Switzerland), the LiteGait device (LiteGait, Tempe, AZ), and the Gait Trainer 3Biodex Gait Training System (Biodex Medical Systems, Inc, Shirley, NY). The prescription of specific parameters including percent body-weight support, speed of the treadmill, support stiffness, and handrail hold can affect treatment outcomes in hemiparetic patients.[62,63] Thus, there may be significant variability in the application of the BWS gait training system and training protocols between clinical settings. In a study of the effect of treadmill speed used during BWS gait training, the greatest improvement in self-selected walking velocity occurred with fast training speeds,[64] thus training at speeds comparable with normal walking velocity may be more effective than training at lower speeds. Specific objective clinical targets, such as heart rate and perceived exertion, can be achieved and/or monitored during BWSTT locomotor training. Patient ease of use has also been reported, as reflected in a recent study[65] that showed that stable walking using BWSTT, as measured by spatiotemporal gait parameters including cadence, step length, and trunk symmetry, was achieved within a 5-minute walking trial.

BWSTT Gait Training and Poststroke Neuroplasticity

Recent research has focused on determining whether BWSTT has an effect on post-stroke neuroplasticity. A therapeutic benefit by neuroplastic mechanisms is largely predicated on research in spinal cord injury that has shown the malleability of the CNS after injury in response to locomotor training.[66–71] Central pattern generators (CPG), neuronal circuitry located within the spinal cord, produce the coordinated activation of flexor and extensor motoneurons during locomotion[72,73] and segmental reflex pathways control the basic operation of the CPG circuitry responsible for locomotion.[74] However, supraspinal input[75] to the spinal circuitry is essential for both human and animal walking. Locomotor training has been shown to change the excitability of simple reflex pathways as well as more complex circuitry, and adaptation occurs at both spinal and supraspinal levels in animals following spinal lesions.[76] Beneficial therapeutic effects of early sustained locomotor training after both central or peripheral lesions, based on evidence of plasticity of spinal and supraspinal locomotor control mechanisms, has thus been advocated.[77]

Researchers have used various neuroimaging modalities to test the hypothesis that BWSTT may influence poststroke central neuroplasticity. Enzinger and colleagues[78] applied an ankle dorsiflexion functional magnetic resonance imaging paradigm to relate brain activity changes in subjects with chronic stroke to performance gains after 4 weeks of BWSTT gait training. At the end of treatment, walking endurance, as measured by the 2-minute walking distance, improved and clinical performance correlated to an increase in brain activity in the bilateral primary sensorimotor cortices, the cingulate motor areas, and the caudate nuclei bilaterally, and in the thalamus of the affected hemisphere. The investigators concluded that, despite subcortical contributions to gait control, walking improvements secondary to BWSTT gait training were associated with cortical activation changes. Another study used an optical imaging system to evaluate the effect of BWSTT on cortical activation during gait in hemiparetic subjects compared with controls.[79] Treatment with BWSTT in the hemiparetic subjects was associated with changes in activation in the sensorimotor cortex (SMC) that correlated with cadence ($P<.05$). Improvement of asymmetry in SMC activation also correlated with improvement of asymmetric gait ($P<.05$). The investigators concluded that BWSTT might improve the efficacy of SMC function in patients with stroke. Further research is necessary to determine whether poststroke BWSTT therapy has central effects and whether those effects translate into clinically significant change in motor impairment and/or functional mobility outcome measures.

Clinical Efficacy of Poststroke BWSTT Gait Training

Multiple studies have suggested beneficial effects of BWSTT gait training in hemiparetic patients on outcomes including walking speed,[80–83] balance,[81,82] walking capacity,[82–84] motor recovery,[81,82] and patient perception of walking ability.[84] Visitin and colleagues[81] compared the effects of BWSTT gait training (40% weight support) with treadmill gait training without BWS. After 6 weeks of training, the BWSTT group scored significantly higher on functional balance, motor recovery, overground walking speed, and overground walking endurance outcome measures. At 3 months after treatment, the BWSTT group continued to score significantly higher than the control group on walking speed and motor recovery measures. In a study that stratified subjects according to initial overground walking speed, endurance, balance, and motor recovery, Barbeau and Visintin[82] found that 6 weeks of BWSTT training resulted in greater walking speed, endurance, functional balance, and motor recovery change than did gait training without BWS. BWSTT was more beneficial to subjects who were older or had a greater baseline level of gait impairment. A recent study[85] explored which kinematic and kinetic gait parameters were most associated with improved walking speed in hemiparetic subjects who were responsive to a 6-week BWSTT program. Subjects who improved their self-selected walking speeds by greater than 0.08 m/s showed greater increases in terminal stance hip extension, hip flexion power, and intensity of soleus muscle EMG activity during walking.

Although beneficial effects have been reported, a Cochrane Review[86] and several recent randomized controlled trials[87–90] show that the superiority of BWSTT gait training compared with standard-of-care gait training interventions has not been established. In a study that compared BWSTT with conventional overground gait training in nonambulatory subacute (<6 weeks after stroke) subjects who had had strokes, Franceschini and colleagues[87] reported that walking speed and capacity, functional ambulation performance, and balance were significantly improved in both groups at the end of 4 weeks of treatment and at the 6-month follow-up. Nilsson and colleagues[89] similarly found no statistically significant difference in Functional Independence Measure score, walking speed, Fugl-Meyer score, and the Berg Balance score gains at end of treatment and at the 10-month follow-up in acute/subacute subjects who hah had strokes randomized to receive either BWSTT or over-ground walking training. More recently, Duncan and colleagues[90] reported on the Locomotor Experience Applied Poststroke (LEAPS) trial, which is the largest study to date to evaluate the efficacy of BWSTT for poststroke gait training. The LEAPS trial enrolled 408 subjects who had had subacute hemiparetic strokes (<2 months after cerebrovascular accident) and stratified the subjects by level of walking impairment. The subjects were then randomized into 1 of 3 gait training groups: (1) BWSTT starting at 2 months after stroke (early locomotor training); (2) BWSTT starting at 6 months after stroke (late locomotor training); and (3) home exercise program (home exercise) starting at 2 months after stroke. The primary outcome measure was the proportion of subjects who had improved functional walking ability at 1 year after stroke. At 1 year, all 3 groups had similar improvements in walking speed, motor recovery, balance, functional status, and quality of life. The investigators concluded that gait training that included the use of BWSTT was not superior to progressive exercise at home managed by a physical therapist. Based on current evidence, Dobkin and Duncan[91] recently concluded that BWSTT does not lead to better outcomes than a comparable dose of progressive overground training after a stroke and should not be routinely provided to stroke survivors in place of conventional therapy.

Summary

BWSTT is a gait training modality that allows otherwise nonambulatory or limited ambulatory patients who have had hemiparetic strokes to participate in task-specific gait training. BWSTT gait training allows a hemiparetic patient to safely weight bear with limited physical assistance while the treating physical therapist focuses on optimizing the gait pattern. BWSTT systems are available for clinical use and are routinely incorporated into poststroke clinical gait training programs. Research supports a beneficial effect of BWSTT on hemiparetic walking speed and capacity, functional balance, and poststroke functional ambulation. Current research is focused on both identifying a neuroplastic mechanism that may explain a therapeutic effect of BWSTT gait training and combining BWS methods with other rehabilitation modalities, such as FES,[92] to maximize poststroke gait rehabilitation outcomes. However, recent randomized controlled clinical trials have not established the superiority of BWSTT compared with other conventional poststroke gait training interventions.

ROBOTIC-ASSISTED GAIT TRAINING FOR HEMIPARESIS

Clinical outpatient stroke rehabilitation programs are increasingly incorporating robotic devices for poststroke gait training. Robotic-assisted gait training involves the use of a powered robot exoskeleton to facilitate repetitive, prolonged, and uniform lower extremity joint and limb movement. Most robotic devices for gait training incorporate some form of body weight support. Although the Lokomat System (Hocoma, Zurich, Switzerland), which combines a robotic orthosis with a body weight support treadmill system, was introduced as a gait training intervention in spinal cord injury in 2003,[93] poststroke gait training using robotic devices was first described as early as the 1990s. Proposed advantages of robotic training include enhanced safety for more severely disabled patients, ability to begin gait training earlier in the poststroke recovery period, increased training time per session, and a decreased physical burden to the treating therapist.[94] Research also suggests that there may be exercise benefits, including improved body tissue composition[95] and improved metabolic and cardiac responses[96] following lower limb robotic gait training. Robots provide the ability to individualize a poststroke gait training program to the specific biomechanical needs of a patient[97] and thus may be efficacious for stroke survivors across a broad spectrum of motor impairment levels.[98] Robotics may be uniquely suited as an early poststroke intervention because of the ability to match task difficulty to patient abilities as motor recovery occurs.[99] In a recent review, Hussain and colleagues[100] described rehabilitation engineering design considerations for treadmill-based robotic gait training devices including type of neurologic injury, level of disability, actuation methods, and training strategies.

Efficacy of Robotic-Assisted Gait Training

Pilot studies have shown improvement in gait velocity,[101–103] 6-minute walking distance,[102,104] balance,[101] motor impairment,[104] spasticity,[104] electromyographic muscle symmetry,[105] and functional ambulation performance[101] associated with a robotic gait training system. Mayr and colleagues[104] reported on a randomized crossover study that enrolled 16 subacute (<3 months) subjects who received robotic gait training alternating with conventional PT for a total of 9 weeks of treatment. Performance on the EU-Walking Scale, Rivermead Motor Assessment Scale, 6-minute walking distance, Medical Research Council Scale (motor strength), and Ashworth Scale (spasticity) was significantly more improved during the robotic training phase than during the conventional treatment phase within each 3-week interval. In a more recent observational study, Conesa and colleagues[101] reported that 80% of 103 subacute inpatient subjects who had had strokes and who received 4 weeks of robotic gait training followed by 4 weeks of manual gait training improved walking speed by more than 0.2 m/s and increased at least 1 point on the Functional Ambulation Category. A recent review of robotic-assisted gait training in neurologic injury also supports that locomotor training with robotic assistance is beneficial for improving walking function in individuals following a stroke.[106]

Robotic-Assisted Gait Training Compared with Conventional Therapy

Several randomized clinical trials[107–111] have suggested that robotic training is better than conventional gait training. In a study of 67 subacute (<3 months) patients who had had strokes randomized to 6 weeks of robotic-assisted gait training or conventional PT,[110] the robotic group showed greater gains in both the National Institute of Health Stroke Scale score and the ability to walk independently at the end of treatment. Stroke survivors with greater motor impairments may benefit more from robotic therapy. Morone and colleagues[108] stratified 48 subacute subjects who had had strokes into 2 motor impairment groups and then randomized them to receive either 3 months of robotic-assisted training (20 sessions) plus conventional therapy, or conventional gait training alone. The lower motricity group who received robotic training showed significant improvement in the Functional Ambulation category, Rivermead Mobility Index, and the 6-minute walking distance, whereas, in the higher motricity groups, robotic and conventional therapies were equivalent. In a follow-up analysis,[109] the greater efficacy of the robotic-assisted program observed in patients with greater motor impairment was sustained after 2 years. A recent Cochrane Review that evaluated 8 trials (414 subjects) concluded that stroke survivors who received robotic-assisted gait training in combination with PT were more likely to achieve independent walking than patients receiving gait training without robotic devices.[112]

In contrast, there are several studies that suggest that poststroke robotic gait training is either no more effective[95,113,114] or less effective than conventional gait training.[115–117] In an early study of 4 weeks of robotic gait training in acute stroke survivors,[95] both the robotic and control groups improved, but there was no significant difference in gait speed or independence between the groups. Fisher[113] randomized 20 stroke survivors to receive either robotic-assisted gait training on a treadmill plus conventional PT versus conventional PT alone. At the end of 24 treatment sessions, both groups showed significant improvement on an 8-m walk test, 3-minute walk test, and the Tinetti Balance Assessment; however, there was no difference between groups. Hornby[116] evaluated the effect of robotic-assisted versus therapist-assisted locomotor training in 48 chronic stroke survivors stratified by level of locomotor deficit. At end of treatment, greater improvement in walking speed and paretic single-stance time was observed in the therapist-assist group. Of 63 subacute (<6 months) stroke survivors randomized to receive either 24 sessions of robotic or conventional gait training,[115] those who received conventional training similarly experienced significantly greater gains in walking speed and 6-minute walking distance than those who received robotic training. These differences were noted at the end of treatment and were maintained at 3 months after treatment. The investigators concluded that the diversity of conventional gait training interventions seemed to be more effective than robotic-assisted gait training for improving walking ability. Dobkin and Duncan[91] recently concluded that current evidence does not support that robotic-assisted step training leads to better poststroke mobility outcomes than a comparable dose of overground gait training and recommend that robotic gait therapy should not be routinely provided in place of conventional therapy.

Robotic-Assisted Therapy Plus Virtual Reality for Gait Training

The efficacy of combining lower extremity robotics with virtual reality to improve gait has been evaluated.[118–122] Forrester[118] reported on 8 chronic stroke survivors who were trained in dorsiflexion and plantarflexion movement by playing video games with a robotic ankle device. At the end of the 6-week training period, improvements were noted in paretic ankle control, walking speed, and single and double support times. Mirelman[120] randomized 18 stroke survivors to receive robotic gait training or robotic gait training combined with virtual reality stimulation. At the end of 4 weeks of training, the virtual reality group showed a significantly larger increase in ankle power generation at push-off,[120] change in ankle range of motion,[120] walking speed,[121] distance walked,[121] and community ambulation.[121] The differences noted in spatiotemporal performance were maintained at 3 months after treatment.[121] The investigators concluded that lower extremity robotic training coupled with virtual reality improved walking ability in stroke survivors and was superior to robotic training alone. Further dose-matched randomized clinical trials that enroll a larger number of subjects are indicated to compare the efficacy of poststroke robotic-assisted gait training with virtual reality with conventional gait therapy.

Summary

Robotic-assisted gait training is a modality that provides repetitive, prolonged, and uniform lower extremity joint and limb movement. Robotic gait training generally incorporates some form of body weight support. Robotic-assisted gait training systems are being investigated in research applications and are increasingly being incorporated into poststroke clinical gait training programs. Research supports beneficial effects of robots on hemiparetic walking speed, walking distance, and functional performance. However, randomized controlled clinical trials have not established the superiority of robotic-assisted gait training compared with other conventional poststroke gait training interventions. In addition, current rehabilitation engineering research is focused on robotic design considerations including improving the patient-machine robotic interface and combining robotics with other modalities, including virtual reality, to maximize poststroke mobility outcomes.

SUMMARY

Maximizing lower extremity motor recovery and functional mobility following stroke is a primary goal for all hemiparetic stroke survivors participating in stroke rehabilitation programs. This article provides a comprehensive overview of the evidence-based research that both supports and disputes the efficacy of lower extremity FES, BWSTT, and robotic-assisted gait training for the treatment of hemiparetic gait. All 3 interventions, which have been trialed extensively in both research and clinical settings, show a positive effect on various gait parameters and measures of walking performance; however, more evidence is necessary to determine whether specific technology-enhanced gait training methods are superior to conventional gait training methods. In addition, further research is necessary to determine how available gait training technologies can be tailored to the specific gait characteristics of the patient. Future studies should focus on evidence of a peripheral and/or central mechanism underlying the therapeutic or compensatory effect of these interventions to further facilitate translation of these technology-based therapies into the clinical care of patients.

REFERENCES

1. Lee RG, van Donkelaar P. Mechanisms underlying functional recovery following stroke. Can J Neurol Sci 1995;22:257–63.
2. Moe JH, Post HW. Functional electrical stimulation for ambulation in hemiplegia. J Lancet 1962;82:285–8.
3. Sheffler LR, Chae J. Neuromuscular electrical stimulation in neurorehabilitation. Muscle Nerve 2007;35:562–90.
4. Mortimer JT. Motor prostheses. In: Brookhart JM, Mountcastle VB, editors. Handbook of physiology-the nervous system II. Bethesda (MD): American Physiological Society; 1981. p. 155–87.
5. Henneman E. Relation between size of neurons and their susceptibility to discharge. Science 1957;126:1345–7.

6. Szlavik RB, de Bruin H. The effect of stimulus current pulse width on nerve fiber size recruitment patterns. Med Eng Phys 1999;21:507–15.
7. Adrian E. The physical background of perception. Oxford (United Kingdom): Clarendon Press; 1946.
8. Kugelberg E, Edstrom L. Differential histochemical effects of muscle contractions on phosphorylase and glycogen in various types of fibres: relation to fatigue. J Neurol Neurosurg Psychiatry 1968;31:415–23.
9. McNeal DR. Analysis of a model for excitation of myelinated nerve. IEEE Trans Biomed Eng 1976;23:329–37.
10. Bigland-Ritchie B, Jones DA, Woods JJ. Excitation frequency and muscle fatigue: electrical responses during human voluntary and stimulated contractions. Exp Neurol 1979;64:414–27.
11. Memberg W, Peckham PH, Keith MH. A surgically implanted intramuscular electrode for an implantable neuromuscular stimulation system. IEEE Trans Biomed Eng 1994;2:80–91.
12. Smith BT, Betz RR, Mulcahey MJ, et al. Reliability of percutaneous intramuscular electrodes for upper extremity functional neuromuscular stimulation in adolescents with C5 tetraplegia. Arch Phys Med Rehabil 1994;75:939–45.
13. Knutson JS, Naples GG, Peckham PH, et al. Electrode fracture rate and occurrences of infection and granuloma associated with percutaneous intramuscular electrodes in upper-limb functional electrical stimulation application. J Rehabil Res Dev 2003;39:671–84.
14. Memberg WD, Peckham PH, Thorpe GB, et al. An analysis of the reliability of percutaneous intramuscular electrodes in upper extremity FNS applications. IEEE Trans Rehabil Eng 1993;1:126–32.
15. Grandjean PA, Mortimer JT. Recruitment properties of monopolar and bipolar epimysial electrodes. Ann Biomed Eng 1986;14:53–66.
16. Waters RL, Campbell JM, Nakai R. Therapeutic electrical stimulation of the lower limb by epimysial electrodes. Clin Orthop Relat Res 1988;233:44–52.
17. Kilgore KL, Peckham PH, Keith MW, et al. Durability of implanted electrodes and leads in an upper-limb neuroprosthesis. J Rehabil Res Dev 2003;40: 457–68.
18. Uhlir JP, Triolo RJ, Kobetic R. The use of selective electrical stimulation of the quadriceps to improve standing function in paraplegia. IEEE Trans Rehabil Eng 2000;8:514–22.
19. Bowman BR, Erickson RC 2nd. Acute and chronic implantation of coiled wire intraneural electrodes during cyclical electrical stimulation. Ann Biomed Eng 1985;13:75–93.
20. Hoffer JA, Loeb GE. Implantable electrical and mechanical interfaces with nerve and muscle. Ann Biomed Eng 1980;8:351–60.
21. Nannini N, Horch K. Muscle recruitment with intrafascicular electrodes. IEEE Trans Biomed Eng 1991;38:769–76.
22. Juch PJ, Minkels RF. The strap-electrode: a stimulating and recording electrode for small nerves. Brain Res Bull 1989;22:917–8.
23. Naples GG, Mortimer JT, Scheiner A, et al. A spiral nerve cuff electrode for peripheral nerve stimulation. IEEE Trans Biomed Eng 1988;35:905–16.
24. Stein RB, Nichols TR, Jhamandas J, et al. Stable long-term recordings from cat peripheral nerves. Brain Res 1977;128:21–38.
25. Sweeney JD, Mortimer JT. An asymmetric two electrode cuff for generation of unidirectionally propagated action potentials. IEEE Trans Biomed Eng 1986; 33:541–9.

26. Kottink AI, Hermens HJ, Nene AV, et al. Therapeutic effect of an implantable peroneal nerve stimulator in subjects with chronic stroke and footdrop: a randomized controlled trial. Phys Ther 2008;88:437–48.

27. Kottink AI, Hermens HJ, Nene AV, et al. A randomized controlled trial of an implantable 2-channel peroneal nerve stimulator on walking speed and activity in poststroke hemiplegia. Arch Phys Med Rehabil 2007;88:971–8.

28. Kottink AI, Tenniglo MJ, de Vries WH, et al. Effects of an implantable two-channel peroneal nerve stimulator versus conventional walking device on spatiotemporal parameters and kinematics of hemiparetic gait. J Rehabil Med 2012;44:51–7.

29. Burridge JH, Taylor PN, Hagan SA, et al. The effects of common peroneal stimulation on the effort and speed of walking: a randomized controlled trial with chronic hemiplegic patients. Clin Rehabil 1997;11:201–10.

30. Dai R, Stein RB, Andrews BJ, et al. Application of tilt sensors in functional electrical stimulation. IEEE Trans Rehabil Eng 1996;4:63–72.

31. Shimada Y, Ando S, Matsunaga T, et al. Clinical application of acceleration sensor to detect the swing phase of stroke gait in functional electrical stimulation. Tohoku J Exp Med 2005;207:197–202.

32. Lieberson W, Holmquest H, Scot D, et al. Functional electrotherapy: stimulation of the peroneal nerve synchronized with the swing phase of the gait of hemiplegia patients. Arch Phys Med Rehabil 1961;42:101–5.

33. Taylor PN, Burridge JH, Dunkerley AL, et al. Clinical use of the Odstock Dropped Foot Stimulator: its effect on the speed and effort of walking. Arch Phys Med Rehabil 1999;80:1577–83.

34. Stein RB, Everaert DG, Thompson AK, et al. Long-term therapeutic and orthotic effects of a foot drop stimulator on walking performance in progressive and nonprogressive neurological disorders. Neurorehabil Neural Repair 2010;24:152–67.

35. Kottink AI, Oostendorp LJ, Buurke JH, et al. The orthotic effect of functional electrical stimulation on the improvement of walking in stroke patients with a dropped foot: a systematic review. Artif Organs 2004;28:577–86.

36. Sheffler LR, Hennessey MT, Naples GG, et al. Improvement in functional ambulation as a therapeutic effect of peroneal nerve stimulation in hemiplegia: two case reports. Neurorehabil Neural Repair 2007;21:366–9.

37. Mann GE, Wright PA, Swain ID. Training effects of electrical stimulation and the conventional ankle foot orthosis in the correction of drop foot following stroke. In: 1st Annual Conference of FESnet 2002. Glasgow (Scotland), 2002.

38. Sabut SK, Sikdar C, Mondal R, et al. Restoration of gait and motor recovery by functional electrical stimulation therapy in persons with stroke. Disabil Rehabil 2010;32:1594–603.

39. Carnstam B, Larsson LE, Prevec TS. Improvement of gait following functional electrical stimulation. I. Investigations on changes in voluntary strength and proprioceptive reflexes. Scand J Rehabil Med 1977;9:7–13.

40. Merletti R, Zelaschi F, Latella D, et al. A control study of muscle force recovery in hemiparetic patients during treatment with functional electrical stimulation. Scand J Rehabil Med 1978;10:147–54.

41. Yan T, Hui-Chan CW, Li LS. Functional electrical stimulation improves motor recovery of the lower extremity and walking ability of subjects with first acute stroke: a randomized placebo-controlled trial. Stroke 2005;36:80–5.

42. Burridge J, Taylor P, Hagan S, et al. Experience of clinical use of the Odstock Dropped Foot Stimulator. Artif Organs 1997;21:254–60.

43. Ring H, Treger I, Gruendlinger L, et al. Neuroprosthesis for footdrop compared with an ankle-foot orthosis: effects on postural control during walking. J Stroke Cerebrovasc Dis 2009;18:41–7.
44. van Swigchem R, van Duijnhoven HJ, den Boer J, et al. Effect of peroneal electrical stimulation versus an ankle-foot orthosis on obstacle avoidance ability in people with stroke-related foot drop. Phys Ther 2012;92:398–406.
45. Waters R, McNeal D, Perry J. Experimental correction of footdrop by electrical stimulation of the peroneal nerve. J Bone Joint Surg Am 1975;57:1047–54.
46. Kljajic M, Malezic M, Acimovic R, et al. Gait evaluation in hemiparetic patients using subcutaneous peroneal electrical stimulation. Scand J Rehabil Med 1992;24:121–6.
47. Kenney L, Bultstra G, Buschman R, et al. An implantable two channel drop foot stimulator: initial clinical results. Artif Organs 2002;26:267–70.
48. Burridge J, Haugland M, Larsen B, et al. A phase II study to evaluate the safety and effectiveness of the ActiGait implanted drop-foot stimulator in established hemiplegia. J Rehabil Med 2007;39(3):212–8.
49. Bogataj U, Gros N, Kljajic M, et al. The rehabilitation of gait in patients with hemiplegia: a comparison between conventional therapy and multichannel functional electrical stimulation therapy. Phys Ther 1995;75:490–502.
50. Bogataj U, Gros N, Malezic M, et al. Restoration of gait during two to three weeks of therapy with multichannel electrical stimulation. Phys Ther 1989;69:319–27.
51. Stanic U, Acimovic-Janezic R, Gros N, et al. Multichannel electrical stimulation for correction of hemiplegic gait. Methodology and preliminary results. Scand J Rehabil Med 1978;10:75–92.
52. Daly JJ, Ruff RL, Haycook K, et al. Feasibility of gait training for acute stroke patients using FNS with implanted electrodes. J Neurol Sci 2000;179:103–7.
53. Daly JJ, Roenigk K, Holcomb J, et al. A randomized controlled trial of functional neuromuscular stimulation in chronic stroke subjects. Stroke 2006;37:172–8 [Epub 2005 Dec 1].
54. Lauer RT, Peckham PH, Kilgore KL, et al. Applications of cortical signals to neuroprosthetic control: a critical review. IEEE Trans Rehabil Eng 2000;8:205–8.
55. Wolpaw JR, Birbaumer N, McFarland DJ, et al. Brain-computer interfaces for communication and control. Clin Neurophysiol 2002;113:767–91.
56. Peckham PH. Development of networked implantable neuroprostheses. In: Cleveland Functional Electrical Stimulation Center. National Institute of Biomedical Imaging and Bioengineering; 2012.
57. Sousa CO, Barela JA, Prado-Medeiros CL, et al. The use of body weight support on ground level: an alternative strategy for gait training of individuals with stroke. J Neuroeng Rehabil 2009;6:43.
58. Sousa CO, Barela JA, Prado-Medeiros CL, et al. Gait training with partial body weight support during overground walking for individuals with chronic stroke: a pilot study. J Neuroeng Rehabil 2011;8:48.
59. Burgess JK, Weibel GC, Brown DA. Overground walking speed changes when subjected to body weight support conditions for nonimpaired and post stroke individuals. J Neuroeng Rehabil 2010;7:6.
60. Danielsson A, Sunnerhagen KS. Oxygen consumption during treadmill walking with and without body weight support in patients with hemiparesis after stroke and in healthy subjects. Arch Phys Med Rehabil 2000;81:953–7.
61. Hesse S, Konrad M, Uhlenbrock D. Treadmill walking with partial body weight support versus floor walking in hemiparetic subjects. Arch Phys Med Rehabil 1999;80:421–7.

62. Chen G, Patten C. Treadmill training with harness support: selection of parameters for individuals with poststroke hemiparesis. J Rehabil Res Dev 2006;43: 485–98.

63. Chen G, Patten C, Kothari DH, et al. Gait deviations associated with post-stroke hemiparesis: improvement during treadmill walking using weight support, speed, support stiffness, and handrail hold. Gait Posture 2005;22:57–62.

64. Sullivan KJ, Knowlton BJ, Dobkin BH. Step training with body weight support: effect of treadmill speed and practice paradigms on poststroke locomotor recovery. Arch Phys Med Rehabil 2002;83:683–91.

65. Aaslund MK, Helbostad JL, Moe-Nilssen R. Familiarisation to body weight supported treadmill training for patients post-stroke. Gait Posture 2011;34:467–72.

66. Behrman AL, Bowden MG, Nair PM. Neuroplasticity after spinal cord injury and training: an emerging paradigm shift in rehabilitation and walking recovery. Phys Ther 2006;86:1406–25.

67. Perez MA, Field-Fote EC, Floeter MK. Patterned sensory stimulation induces plasticity in reciprocal Ia inhibition in humans. J Neurosci 2003;23:2014–8.

68. Frigon A, Rossignol S. Functional plasticity following spinal cord lesions. Prog Brain Res 2006;157:231–60.

69. Scivoletto G, Ivanenko Y, Morganti B, et al. Plasticity of spinal centers in spinal cord injury patients: new concepts for gait evaluation and training. Neurorehabil Neural Repair 2007;21:358–65.

70. Wolpaw JR. The education and re-education of the spinal cord. Prog Brain Res 2006;157:261–80.

71. Wolpaw JR. Spinal cord plasticity in acquisition and maintenance of motor skills. Acta Physiol (Oxf) 2007;189:155–69.

72. McCrea DA, Rybak IA. Organization of mammalian locomotor rhythm and pattern generation. Brain Res Rev 2008;57(1):134–46.

73. Dietz V. Spinal cord pattern generators for locomotion. Clin Neurophysiol 2003; 114:1379–89.

74. McCrea DA. Spinal circuitry of sensorimotor control of locomotion. J Physiol 2001;533:41–50.

75. Rossignol S, Dubuc R, Gossard JP. Dynamic sensorimotor interactions in locomotion. Physiol Rev 2006;86:89–154.

76. Rossignol S. Plasticity of connections underlying locomotor recovery after central and/or peripheral lesions in the adult mammals. Philos Trans R Soc Lond B Biol Sci 2006;361:1647–71.

77. Rossignol S, Brustein E, Bouyer L, et al. Adaptive changes of locomotion after central and peripheral lesions. Can J Physiol Pharmacol 2004;82:617–27.

78. Enzinger C, Dawes H, Johansen-Berg H, et al. Brain activity changes associated with treadmill training after stroke. Stroke 2009;40:2460–7.

79. Miyai I, Suzuki M, Hatakenaka M, et al. Effect of body weight support on cortical activation during gait in patients with stroke. Exp Brain Res 2006;169:85–91.

80. Hesse S, Bertelt C, Jahnke MT, et al. Treadmill training with partial body weight support compared with physiotherapy in nonambulatory hemiparetic patients. Stroke 1995;26:976–81.

81. Visintin M, Barbeau H, Korner-Bitensky N, et al. A new approach to retrain gait in stroke patients through body weight support and treadmill stimulation. Stroke 1998;29:1122–8.

82. Barbeau H, Visintin M. Optimal outcomes obtained with body-weight support combined with treadmill training in stroke subjects. Arch Phys Med Rehabil 2003;84:1458–65.

83. Sullivan KJ, Brown DA, Klassen T, et al. Effects of task-specific locomotor and strength training in adults who were ambulatory after stroke: results of the STEPS randomized clinical trial. Phys Ther 2007;87:1580–602.

84. Dean CM, Ada L, Bampton J, et al. Treadmill walking with body weight support in subacute non-ambulatory stroke improves walking capacity more than overground walking: a randomised trial. J Physiother 2010;56:97–103.

85. Mulroy SJ, Klassen T, Gronley JK, et al. Gait parameters associated with responsiveness to treadmill training with body-weight support after stroke: an exploratory study. Phys Ther 2010;90:209–23.

86. Moseley AM, Stark A, Cameron ID, et al. Treadmill training and body weight support for walking after stroke. Cochrane Database Syst Rev 2005;(4):CD002840.

87. Franceschini M, Carda S, Agosti M, et al. Walking after stroke: what does treadmill training with body weight support add to overground gait training in patients early after stroke? A single-blind, randomized, controlled trial. Stroke 2009;40: 3079–85.

88. Hoyer E, Jahnsen R, Stanghelle JK, et al. Body weight supported treadmill training versus traditional training in patients dependent on walking assistance after stroke: a randomized controlled trial. Disabil Rehabil 2012;34:210–9.

89. Nilsson L, Carlsson J, Danielsson A, et al. Walking training of patients with hemiparesis at an early stage after stroke: a comparison of walking training on a treadmill with body weight support and walking training on the ground. Clin Rehabil 2001;15:515–27.

90. Duncan PW, Sullivan KJ, Behrman AL, et al. Body-weight-supported treadmill rehabilitation after stroke. N Engl J Med 2011;364:2026–36.

91. Dobkin BH, Duncan PW. Should body weight-supported treadmill training and robotic-assistive steppers for locomotor training trot back to the starting gate? Neurorehabil Neural Repair 2012;26:308–17.

92. Prado-Medeiros CL, Sousa CO, Souza AS, et al. Effects of the addition of functional electrical stimulation to ground level gait training with body weight support after chronic stroke. Rev Bras Fisioter 2011;15:436–44.

93. Jezernik S, Colombo G, Keller T, et al. Robotic orthosis Lokomat: a rehabilitation and research tool. Neuromodulation 2003;6:108–15.

94. Sayers SP, Krug J. Robotic gait-assisted therapy in patients with neurological injury. Mo Med 2008;105:153–8.

95. Husemann B, Muller F, Krewer C, et al. Effects of locomotion training with assistance of a robot-driven gait orthosis in hemiparetic patients after stroke: a randomized controlled pilot study. Stroke 2007;38:349–54.

96. Hidler J, Hamm LF, Lichy A, et al. Automating activity-based interventions: the role of robotics. J Rehabil Res Dev 2008;45:337–44.

97. Koenig A, Omlin X, Bergmann J, et al. Controlling patient participation during robot-assisted gait training. J Neuroeng Rehabil 2011;8:14.

98. Huang VS, Krakauer JW. Robotic neurorehabilitation: a computational motor learning perspective. J Neuroeng Rehabil 2009;6:5.

99. Colombo R, Sterpi I, Mazzone A, et al. Taking a lesson from patients' recovery strategies to optimize training during robot-aided rehabilitation. IEEE Trans Neural Syst Rehabil Eng 2012;20:276–85.

100. Hussain S, Xie SQ, Liu G. Robot assisted treadmill training: mechanisms and training strategies. Med Eng Phys 2011;33:527–33.

101. Conesa L, Costa U, Morales E, et al. An observational report of intensive robotic and manual gait training in sub-acute stroke. J Neuroeng Rehabil 2012;9:13.

102. Wu M, Landry JM, Yen SC, et al. A novel cable-driven robotic training improves locomotor function in individuals post-stroke. Conf Proc IEEE Eng Med Biol Soc 2011;2011:8539–42.
103. Westlake KP, Patten C. Pilot study of Lokomat versus manual-assisted treadmill training for locomotor recovery post-stroke. J Neuroeng Rehabil 2009;6:18.
104. Mayr A, Kofler M, Quirbach E, et al. Prospective, blinded, randomized crossover study of gait rehabilitation in stroke patients using the Lokomat gait orthosis. Neurorehabil Neural Repair 2007;21:307–14.
105. Coenen P, van Werven G, van Nunen MP, et al. Robot-assisted walking vs overground walking in stroke patients: an evaluation of muscle activity. J Rehabil Med 2012;44:331–7.
106. Tefertiller C, Pharo B, Evans N, et al. Efficacy of rehabilitation robotics for walking training in neurological disorders: a review. J Rehabil Res Dev 2011; 48:387–416.
107. Hesse S, Tomelleri C, Bardeleben A, et al. Robot-assisted practice of gait and stair climbing in nonambulatory stroke patients. J Rehabil Res Dev 2012;49: 613–22.
108. Morone G, Bragoni M, Iosa M, et al. Who may benefit from robotic-assisted gait training? A randomized clinical trial in patients with subacute stroke. Neurorehabil Neural Repair 2011;25:636–44.
109. Morone G, Iosa M, Bragoni M, et al. Who may have durable benefit from robotic gait training? A 2-year follow-up randomized controlled trial in patients with subacute stroke. Stroke 2012;43:1140–2.
110. Schwartz I, Sajin A, Fisher I, et al. The effectiveness of locomotor therapy using robotic-assisted gait training in subacute stroke patients: a randomized controlled trial. PM R 2009;1:516–23.
111. Chang WH, Kim MS, Huh JP, et al. Effects of robot-assisted gait training on cardiopulmonary fitness in subacute stroke patients: a randomized controlled study. Neurorehabil Neural Repair 2012;26:318–24.
112. Mehrholz J, Werner C, Kugler J, et al. Electromechanical-assisted training for walking after stroke. Cochrane Database Syst Rev 2007;(4):CD006185.
113. Fisher S, Lucas L, Thrasher TA. Robot-assisted gait training for patients with hemiparesis due to stroke. Top Stroke Rehabil 2011;18:269–76.
114. Bogey R, Hornby GT. Gait training strategies utilized in poststroke rehabilitation: are we really making a difference? Top Stroke Rehabil 2007;14:1–8.
115. Hidler J, Nichols D, Pelliccio M, et al. Multicenter randomized clinical trial evaluating the effectiveness of the Lokomat in subacute stroke. Neurorehabil Neural Repair 2009;23:5–13.
116. Hornby TG, Campbell DD, Kahn JH, et al. Enhanced gait-related improvements after therapist- versus robotic-assisted locomotor training in subjects with chronic stroke: a randomized controlled study. Stroke 2008;39:1786–92.
117. Lewek MD, Cruz TH, Moore JL, et al. Allowing intralimb kinematic variability during locomotor training poststroke improves kinematic consistency: a subgroup analysis from a randomized clinical trial. Phys Ther 2009;89:829–39.
118. Forrester LW, Roy A, Krebs HI, et al. Ankle training with a robotic device improves hemiparetic gait after a stroke. Neurorehabil Neural Repair 2011;25: 369–77.
119. Kim SH, Banala SK, Brackbill EA, et al. Robot-assisted modifications of gait in healthy individuals. Exp Brain Res 2010;202:809–24.
120. Mirelman A, Patritti BL, Bonato P, et al. Effects of virtual reality training on gait biomechanics of individuals post-stroke. Gait Posture 2010;31:433–7.

121. Mirelman A, Bonato P, Deutsch JE. Effects of training with a robot-virtual reality system compared with a robot alone on the gait of individuals after stroke. Stroke 2009;40:169–74.
122. Wellner M, Thuring T, Smajic E, et al. Obstacle crossing in a virtual environment with the rehabilitation gait robot LOKOMAT. Stud Health Technol Inform 2007; 125:497–9.

Ambulation and Multiple Sclerosis

Robert W. Motl, PhD

KEYWORDS

- Walking • Ambulation • Quality of life • Exercise • Disability • Multiple sclerosis

KEY POINTS

- Walking impairment is a prevalent consequence of multiple sclerosis (MS) that is primarily driven by pathologic changes in the central nervous system and can result in substantial limitations of daily activities and compromised quality of life.
- Walking impairments can be used to monitor disability and disease progression in clinical practice and therapeutic trials involving patients with MS.
- Assessments of walking impairment range from gait analysis in the laboratory through monitoring of community ambulation with motion sensors.
- Emerging evidence supports the use of pharmacologic and rehabilitation approaches, particularly exercise training, as effective for improving walking and mobility in patients with MS.

INTRODUCTION

Multiple sclerosis (MS) is a prevalent, nontraumatic, and disabling disease of the central nervous system (CNS) that is most often diagnosed in young and middle-aged individuals (of which two-thirds are women) of European descent. Approximately 2.5 million cases of MS exist worldwide and 400,000 cases have been diagnosed in the United States.[1] MS typically causes areas of inflammation in the CNS[2] that result in axonal demyelination and transection.[3] Neurodegenerative changes seemingly associated with a lack of neurotrophic support further occur over the course of MS.[3] The CNS damage caused by MS manifests in several ways,[4] and impairment of ambulation or walking (ie, over-ground movement by taking steps with one's feet), in particular, represents one of the most common, challenging, and life-altering consequences of MS.[5] This article provides a focused overview on walking impairment, its importance, and its management in persons with MS.

Disclosures: This paper was supported by grants from the National Multiple Sclerosis Society (RG 3926A2/1, RG 4499A3/1, and PP 1695).
Department of Kinesiology and Community Health, University of Illinois at Urbana-Champaign, 233 Freer Hall, Urbana, IL 61801, USA
E-mail address: robmotl@uiuc.edu

Phys Med Rehabil Clin N Am 24 (2013) 325–336
http://dx.doi.org/10.1016/j.pmr.2012.11.004
1047-9651/13/$ – see front matter

WALKING IMPAIRMENT IN MS
A Common Occurrence

Walking impairment has long been considered a primary feature of MS, even in early historical accounts of the disease.[6] An estimated 75% of persons with MS report mobility problems based on population-based studies.[7] Recent data from an online survey of 1011 people with MS indicated that 41% of the sample reported having difficulty walking and 13% reported an inability to walk.[5] Another recent study of 436 patients with MS in Europe indicated that nearly 1 in 2 patients reported experiencing mobility impairments within the first month of diagnosis, and more than 90% of patients reported experiencing mobility impairments within 10 years of diagnosis.[8] Overall, these data suggest that walking impairment is (1) common in MS, even early in the disease, and (2) a long-term consequence that likely affects most persons living with this neurologic disease.

Primarily Caused by CNS Pathology

The pathology of MS is important in understanding the occurrence of walking impairment in this population. This discussion of pathology and its association with walking is based on an existing conceptual framework derived from the World Health Organization's International Classification of Function.[9] MS is a disease that involves demyelination and axonal transection in the white and gray matter, which results in dysfunction and atrophy within various regions of the CNS, including the pyramidal, cerebellar, and spinal/dorsal column pathways.[3,9] This CNS pathology manifests in impairments such as muscle weakness and spasticity, ataxia, and sensory disturbances.[9] These impairments[10] and those of vision and cognition, along with secondary factors (eg, weight gain, fatigue, or deconditioning),[11] can result in altered gait kinematics and spatial and temporal parameters of gait (base of support, double support, cadence, step length, and velocity),[12] even early in the disease process.[13] The changes in gait kinematics and spatiotemporal parameters alter the normally smooth and rhythmic sinusoidal vertical displacement of the body's center of mass during ambulation (ie, inverted pendulum of gait).[14,15] This disruption ultimately manifests as altered ambulation, quantified via performance tests, physiologic parameters, self-report questionnaires, and free-living assessments.[16]

Important to Persons with MS

Walking is a fundamental part of life and daily existence, regardless of the presence or absence of disease and chronic conditions. Among persons with MS, ambulation represents one of the most valued functions[5,17] and has direct relevance to physical function, independence, quality of life, and activities of daily living.[8,17] For example, one study of 100 patients with MS reported that walking was rated as the most important domain of function compared with 12 other functions, such as vision, thinking and memory, and mood,[18] in both early (<5 years duration) and late (>15 years duration) MS. Of further importance, one study reported that persons with MS described feeling limited, frustrated, powerless, and challenged by mobility impairment.[8] Another study indicated that 70% of persons with MS who had difficulty walking rated it as the most challenging aspect of MS.[5] Walking difficulty has been associated with adverse outcomes regarding employment,[5,19] physical function, quality of life, and activities and participation.[20] For example, one study of 196 persons with MS reported that being unemployed was independently associated with reduced community ambulation based on the metric of steps per day recorded in real life.[19]

Clinically Important

Beyond concerns of personal relevance and importance, ambulatory impairment represents a defining feature of disease progression in MS[21] and is a common component of clinical outcome measures such as the Expanded Disability Status Scale (EDSS)[22] and the Multiple Sclerosis Functional Composite (MSFC).[23] These measures are often included in natural history studies and/or clinical trials in MS.[21-23] The EDSS is a 10-point scale of disease severity ranging between 0 (no disability) and 10 (death from MS). Scores from 0 through 3.5 reflect changes in 1 or more of 8 functional systems, whereas scores 4.0 and greater are based primarily on changes in ambulation (walking distance up to 500 m and the need for assistive devices to walk). Based on the EDSS, natural history studies have examined the rate and predictors of disability progression in persons with MS based on benchmark scores. For example, the median times from onset of MS until the assignment of benchmark EDSS scores of 4.0 (ie, limited walking ability but able to walk more than 500 m without aid or rest) and 6.0 (ie, ability to walk with unilateral support about 100 m without rest) are approximately 10 and 20 years, respectively.[24-26] The MSFC is a new, composite clinical measure based on measurement of ambulation (timed 25-ft walk [T25FW]), upper extremity function (9-hole peg test), and cognition (paced auditory serial addition test), which was developed based on the need for an outcome measure that better reflects progression of disease and clinical change in MS.[23] The T25FW, in particular, has become a prominent stand-alone component for capturing clinically meaningful change in ambulation and disease progression among persons with MS.[27] These assessments, and others, provide important information to clinicians for monitoring the rate of progression of MS over time and the results of treatments.

Performance and Gait Characteristics

The extent and type of walking impairment in MS can be described by considering common outcomes of this functional behavior. For example, 2 of the most common walking performance assessments include the T25FW and 6-minute walk (6MW) as measures of short- and long-distance (or endurance) ambulatory function, respectively.[28] The T25FW involves having a patient walk 25 ft as fast and safe as possible, and the time is recorded in seconds by averaging 2 consecutive trials. The T25FW was recently recognized as the best-characterized objective measure of walking disability in persons with MS across a wide range of walking impairments.[28] Data indicate that performance on the T25FW is compromised in persons with MS compared with controls who do not have MS or any other neurologic disease.[29,30] For example, one study reported that T25FW performance was significantly worse in 141 patients with MS (median, 4.4 seconds) than in 104 healthy controls (median, 3.7 seconds), and the differences in T25FW performance existed across 3 levels of disability (EDSS, 0–2.0; median, 3.9 seconds; EDSS, 2.5–3.5; median, 4.5 seconds; and EDSS, 4.0–5.5, median, 5.8 seconds).[29] Further evidence indicates that a 20% or greater change in T25FW performance is clinically meaningful.[28] Overall, this indicates that compromised walking speed over a short distance is one facet of impaired ambulation in MS, and that a 20% change represents a significant worsening or improvement in one's capacity for ambulation.

The 6MW involves having a person walk as fast and as far as possible during a 6-minute period and the distance is recorded in feet or meters.[30] Consistent data indicate that performance on the 6MW is compromised in persons with MS compared with controls who do not have MS or any other neurologic disease.[30-33] For example, the first application of the 6MW in this population indicated that persons with MS (n = 40) showed a large reduction in 6MW distance (eg, Cohen's effect size d of ~1.4 for first 6MW) compared with matched controls (n = 20), and the 6MW distance further differed between MS subjects who had mild (EDSS, 0–2.5), moderate (EDSS, 3.0–4.0), and severe (EDSS, 4.5–6.5) disability.[30] The effect of disability on 6MW performance was replicated in a larger sample of 95 persons with clinically definite MS.[33] Another study reported a similarly large difference in the 6MW distance (Cohen's effect size d of ~1.5) between persons with MS (n = 33) and age- and sex-matched controls (n = 33).[31] Collectively, this indicates that compromised walking endurance capacity is another manifestation of walking impairment in persons with MS.

The impairments in T25FW and 6MW performance are likely associated with changes in spatial and temporal manifestations of gait, which along with kinematics describe (CIR Systems Inc, Haverton, PA, USA) the mechanics of walking. Spatial and temporal gait parameters were well characterized recently based on data recorded from the GAITRite electronic walkway in persons with MS.[34–37] For example, one study reported that persons with MS (n = 43) who had minimal disability (ie, ambulatory without an assistive device) walked slower (ie, decreased velocity) by taking fewer (decreased cadence), shorter (decreased step length), and wider steps (increased base of support), and spent a greater portion of the gait cycle in double support than controls who were matched on age, height, weight, and sex.[36] Another study reported differences in velocity, cadence, step length and time, double support, and swing phase among persons with MS (n = 78) as a function of disability level (ie, mild, moderate, and severe) based on EDSS scores.[35] Those gait parameters have been associated with changes in ambulation.[12,38] Taken as a whole, this indicates that the gait cycle and its descriptive parameters are compromised in persons with MS and likely contribute to impairments in walking performance.

Physiologic Characteristics

Another way of describing walking impairment that occurs in MS involves physiologic parameters. The oxygen (O_2) cost of walking (ie, milliliters of O_2 consumed per kilogram of body weight per meter traveled [$mL/kg^{-1}/m^{-1}$]) is a physiologic marker that reflects the degree of locomotor impairment in pathologic conditions based on the energetic cost of movement.[39] The O_2 cost of walking reflects either an increase in the rate of O_2 consumption ($\dot{V}O_2$) with normal walking speed (ie, increased energy expenditure for doing the same movement) or a reduction in walking speed with a normal $\dot{V}O_2$ (ie, same energy expenditure for doing less movement). Overall, an increase in the O_2 cost would indicate that walking is more physiologically effortful and less efficient for persons with MS, and this might explain why walking impairment has such a large effect on daily activities and participation in this population.

The examination of physiologic markers during ambulation in MS has been a recent area of interest for researchers.[32,39–43] For example, one study examined the pattern of change in $\dot{V}O_2$ in relation to performance on the 6MW in a large sample of persons with MS (n = 95) with a wide range of disability (median EDSS, 4.5; range, 2.0–6.5).[32] The rate of increase in $\dot{V}O_2$ during the 6MW was steeper in those with mild disability (EDSS, 2.0–3.5) than those with moderate (EDSS, 4.0–5.5) and severe disability (EDSS, 6.0–6.5), and those with mild disability had a higher overall rate of $\dot{V}O_2$ than those with moderate and severe disability. This finding seems counterintuitive but is logical, because those with mild disability walked further with a faster speed and cadence, thereby requiring greater $\dot{V}O_2$ during the 6MW. This pattern illustrates the importance of expressing $\dot{V}O_2$ during walking against speed and/or distance.

Accordingly, other studies have indicated that persons with MS have a higher O_2 cost of walking than matched controls,[40–43] and this differs based on walking impairment[39] and disability status,[41] such that those with worse walking and disability have a higher O_2 cost of walking. The existing data, when taken as a whole, indicate that walking is more physiologically demanding for persons with MS, particularly as a function of increasing levels of disability and walking impairment.

Free-Living Assessments

Walking impairments in MS have often been documented based on assessments performed in a laboratory or clinical setting. These measurements are accurate, reliable, and valid, but lack ecologic validity for understanding ambulation that occurs in the context of daily life.[16] Accordingly, another way of describing walking impairments in MS involves assessing ambulation in free-living conditions using accelerometers and pedometers. These devices are motion sensors, often worn around the waist near the center of mass, and capture the vertical displacement of the body during ambulatory activity undertaken in the real world during the waking hours of the day without disrupting normal activities. The changes in this community ambulation are driven by changes in performance, gait pattern, and physiologic manifestations of walking in MS.[12,16,38]

Consistent evidence indicates reduced community ambulation in persons with MS based on motion sensor data.[20,44–46] For example, one study reported a large difference (Cohen's effect size d of ~1.0) in activity counts per day from a waist-worn Acti-Graph accelerometer between persons with MS (n = 33) and a matched control sample (n = 33), indicating that the persons with MS were engaging in less community-based ambulation.[46] This finding has been replicated in other research involving samples with MS and age-, sex-, height-, and weight-matched controls.[44] The authors further note that impaired community ambulation is directly associated with disability status based on the EDSS in persons with MS.[20,45] For example, one study reported a linear reduction in activity counts per day from a waist-worn Acti-Graph accelerometer as a function of increasing disability (mild: EDSS, 0–3.5; moderate: EDSS, 4.0–5.5; and severe: EDSS ≥6.0) and differences based on ambulatory status classified by assistive device use in a sample of 70 persons with MS.[45] The effect of disability status has been confirmed in other research using the Step-Watch Step Activity Monitor and metric of steps per day in persons with MS.[20] These reductions in activity and step counts suggest that walking impairment extends beyond the laboratory and into the community, thereby affecting one's ambulation as part of everyday life.

Coupling with Cognition

An exciting new area of research involves examining the coupling of walking and thinking. This interest is based, in part, on the recognition that walking is not simply an automated motor behavior but rather a complex behavior with multifaceted neuropsychological influences,[47] especially because persons with MS must make a conscious effort to walk safely despite increasing neurologic impairments. This research is further based on the idea that the extent of walking impairment can be exaggerated when performing a second task that stresses or overloads one's neural systems. Indeed, considerable overlap exists in regions of the brain associated with walking and thinking, and MS often affects these areas.[48] Therefore, competition exists for the same regions of the brain (ie, neural resources), and performing a cognitive task while walking should be associated with worse performance than when simply walking alone.

One of the first studies of cognitive–motor coupling in MS examined the association between neuropsychological performance (ie, processing speed and executive function) and lower-extremity performance based on the T25FW in 211 patients with MS and 120 healthy volunteers. Associations were seen between cognition and T25FW performance in persons with MS and controls, although the associations were more robust in the MS sample. Further associations were seen between cognitive and T25FW performance in the MS sample, even after controlling for confounders, including disease duration and disability status based on EDSS.[48] This coupling was more recently demonstrated after having patients undertake a cognitive task while walking, and then examining the effect of the combined tasks versus walking alone on gait outcomes. This process and outcome has been termed the *dual-task cost* (DTC) of walking. One study reported an overall decline in gait with an additive cognitive task, with a range in DTC of 1.8% for step length through 12% for gait velocity in 78 persons with clinically definite MS.[35] The DTC was significantly larger in persons with moderate (n = 25; EDSS, 4.0–5.5) and severe (n = 32; EDSS, 6.0–6.5) disability compared with those who had mild disability (n = 21; EDSS, 2.0–3.5).[35] Additional data indicate that the DTC of walking is greater in persons with MS (n = 18) than in healthy controls (n = 18),[49] and this detriment in walking while thinking has even been observed in persons with early MS (52 patients with clinically isolated syndrome) versus age- and sex-matched controls (n = 28).[50] This problem with walking and thinking in MS might have practical implications for everyday activities that require cognition and ambulation (eg, walking across a busy street), and could further result in adverse events during ambulation, such as falling.

MANAGEMENT OF WALKING IMPAIRMENTS IN MS
Pharmacologic Approach

The prevalence, clinical and personal relevance, and extent of walking impairment from the laboratory into the real world underscore the importance of managing this consequence of MS. One exciting pharmacologic approach for managing walking impairment in MS involves oral administration of dalfampridine (extended-release 4-aminopyridine [4-AP], also called *fampridine*). This pharmacologic approach has been the topic of recent literature reviews.[51,52] 4-AP is a potassium channel blocker that can increase action potential duration and amplitude, and therefore improve conduction in demyelinated nerves and neurotransmitter release at synaptic endings (although this has been demonstrated only in vitro).

Recently, the effect of 4-AP on ambulation, based on the T25FW and Multiple Sclerosis Walking Scale-12 (MSWS-12), was tested in a phase III multicenter, randomized, controlled, double-blind study of persons with MS who underwent 14 weeks of treatment with oral sustained-release 4-AP at 10-mg twice-daily, or placebo.[53] A higher proportion of "timed walk responders" (ie, subjects who exhibited consistent improvement on T25FW during on-treatment visits compared with off-treatment visits) was seen in the fampridine (35%) than in the placebo (8%) group, and this was further supported by improvements in MSWS-12 scores. These positive results were replicated in a subsequent phase III trial.[54] This research supports oral sustained-release 4-AP as the first symptomatic pharmaceutical treatment approved for the treatment of walking impairment in MS, based on improved walking speed in clinical trials. Other symptomatic therapies for MS, such as treatments for spasticity and neuropathic pain, may have an impact on walking and mobility in persons with MS but have not been well studied for this particular outcome.[55] Disease-modifying therapies (eg, interferon beta, glatiramer acetate, natalizumab, or fingolimod) can slow the rate of disability progression (and hence ambulatory impairment) over long periods[24–26] but do not currently represent an approach for directly restoring or improving ambulation in persons with MS.

Exercise as a Behavioral Approach

Beyond pharmaceuticals, many rehabilitation or behavioral approaches are available for managing walking impairment in persons with MS. Most research studies have focused on exercise training as a behavioral approach for improving walking. Exercise training refers to prescribed physical activity behavior undertaken in a repetitive structured routine over a prolonged period with a goal of improving fitness, symptoms, or function. Recent literature reviews[56–58] have summarized the existing research on exercise training and its influence on walking in MS.

Furthermore, a recent meta-analysis examined the effect of exercise training on walking mobility among persons with MS.[59] This involved a search for published exercise training studies from 1960 to November 2007, using MEDLINE, PsychINFO, CINAHL, and CURRENT CONTENTS PLUS. Forty-three published papers were located and reviewed, and 22 provided enough data to compute effect sizes expressed as Cohen's d. Sixty-six effect sizes were retrieved from the 22 publications with 609 MS participants and yielded a weighted mean effect size (Hedge's g) of 0.19 (95% CI, 0.09, 0.28). The cumulative evidence supported that exercise training was associated with a small improvement in walking mobility among individuals with MS, but most studies have been conducted in samples with minimal disability rather than among those at later stages of MS who have sustained walking impairment.

Accordingly, one recently completed study examined a combined exercise training stimulus and its influence on a comprehensive set of walking outcomes in persons with EDSS scores between 4.0 and 6.0.[60] Participants (N = 13; EDSS range, 4.0–6.0) completed the MSWS-12; 2 trials of the T25FW and Timed Up and Go (TUG) test; and 4 walking trials on a 26-foot GAITRite (CIR Systems, Inc, Haverton, PA, USA) before and after an 8-week training period. The exercise training program was supervised by an exercise specialist and consisted of aerobic, resistance, and balance training performed 3 days per week. The duration of exercise was initially 15 minutes a week 1 (ie, 5 minutes of each mode of exercise) and increased by approximately 5 minutes per week up to a maximum of 60 minutes in week 8 (ie, 20 minutes of each mode of exercise). Improvements were seen in MSWS-12 scores, T25FW and TUG performance, and Functional Ambulation Profile score from the GAITRite. These results suggest that a combined exercise training stimulus represents a comprehensive physiologically relevant rehabilitation strategy that is associated with improved walking mobility in persons with MS who have onset of gait impairment.

Some researchers have examined the effects of assisted exercise training on walking performance in persons with advanced MS. This type of training includes body weight–supported treadmill training (BWSTT) and robot-assisted locomotor training, either individually or together, in persons with progressive MS and severe disability.[61–64] Walking speed and endurance have improved significantly after robot-assisted treadmill training in persons with MS with gait impairment,[61,63] and this may be a function of the task-specific nature of the training modality.[58] The improvement was observed after 15 sessions of BWSTT with the Lokomat robotic device in a sample of 14 persons with MS who had median EDSS scores of 6.5 (range, 6.0–7.6),[61] and after 6 training sessions of BWSTT with or without Lokomat in a sample of 13 persons with MS who had mean EDSS scores of 4.9 (SD, 1.2).[63]

Beyond exercise training, inpatient and outpatient rehabilitation approaches involving physiotherapy have been effective for improving walking in persons with MS.[65,66] Unfortunately, the rehabilitation interventions are often not described in detail in these studies, and the outcome measures used are not consistent across studies. Of note, Vaney and colleagues[67] found that robot-assisted gait training was not superior to traditional over-ground gait training in a randomized controlled trial involving 67 patients with MS and an EDSS score between 3.0 and 6.5. Rehabilitation technology might also be effective for improving walking in persons with MS,[65] including ankle-foot or hip orthoses for managing balance, muscle weakness, and/or ambulatory impairment, and functional electrical stimulation as an approach to overcoming foot drop in persons with MS.

FUTURE RESEARCH

Considering the existing literature, a tremendous amount of research obviously can be undertaken to increase understanding of walking impairment and its management in MS. One of the most obvious future directions involves examining the independent, interactive, and additive effects of exercise training and pharmaceutical approaches.[57,58] These approaches might work through different mechanisms of action, thereby resulting in additive effects on ambulation. For example, exercise training could result in a positive adaptation of brain structure and function[68,69] or physiologic conditioning,[56,57] whereas 4-AP seemingly works through an increase in action potential duration and amplitude, an improvement of conduction in demyelinated nerves, and neurotransmitter release at synaptic endings. Pharmaceutical approaches might allow significantly greater amounts of exercise training, which would yield even larger changes in walking performance.

Another research direction involves focusing on exercise training and other rehabilitation techniques in persons with advanced MS, in whom ambulatory and gait impairment are more pronounced, severe, and restrictive. This undertaking might include further research on the use of BWSTT or robot-assisted locomotor training in persons with progressive MS or severe disability, and might focus on multimodal exercise training combining aerobic exercise, lower-body resistance training, and balance training to comprehensively target physiologic deconditioning as a source of walking impairment in persons with MS who have moderate disability.[57]

Additional research is necessary focusing on other metrics to assess the benefits of therapeutic interventions on walking impairment in persons with MS. For example, exercise training has the potential to impact walking[59] and cognition,[70] and this suggests the possibility of reducing the negative effects of thinking while walking in persons with MS (ie, DTC). Increasing research is focusing on metrics of community ambulation in MS based on accelerometry,[16] and researchers should examine whether the effects of therapeutic interventions extend outside the laboratory (ie, 6MW or T25FW) and into the real world. The findings might be important in improving the capacity of persons with MS to accomplish daily activities, experience community integration, and maintain sustained employment.

Lastly, research should focus on identifying neural imaging-based approaches to promote a better understanding of neural correlates of ambulatory impairment and mechanisms for improved ambulation with therapeutic intervention. For example, functional magnetic resonance imaging has been applied to increase understanding of neural correlates of cognitive processes in older adults,[71] and has been subsequently applied for understanding neural mechanisms of exercise and its effects on cognitive performance.[72] This same paradigm has been adopted for establishing neural mechanisms of fitness, exercise training, and cognition in MS.[67,68] Logically, the development of a similar paradigm would be fruitful for understanding walking impairment and its remediation in MS.

SUMMARY

Walking impairment and loss of ambulation are common consequences of MS that can result in a substantial patient burden in performing daily activities and a compromised quality of life. Walking impairment in persons with MS is primarily driven by pathologic changes in the CNS, and therefore is often monitored as an indicator of disease and neurologic disability progression. Measures of walking impairment range from gait analysis (detecting early changes before they become clinically observable), to performance on standardized tests in the clinic, to real-world metrics (eg, pedometers and oscillometers, and patient-reported outcomes). Researchers have considered pharmaceutical and rehabilitation approaches for managing walking impairment in MS, and both approaches have yielded beneficial effects on walking outcomes, although most research has focused on exercise training. Walking impairment has ubiquitous and life-altering consequences in MS, underscoring the importance of identifying approaches to prevent and forestall this event, and to restore walking ability in persons with MS. This approach holds considerable promise for impacting the lives of persons with MS, and is seemingly a critical goal for clinical research and practice.

REFERENCES

1. National Multiple Sclerosis Society. Multiple sclerosis information sourcebook. New York: Information Resource Center and Library of the National Multiple Sclerosis Society; 2005.
2. Hemmer B, Nessler S, Zhou D, et al. Immunopathogenesis and immunotherapy of multiple sclerosis. Nat Clin Pract Neurol 2006;2:201–11.
3. Trapp BD, Nave K. Multiple sclerosis: an immune or neurodegenerative disorder? Annu Rev Neurosci 2008;31:247–69.
4. Lublin FD. Clinical features and diagnosis of multiple sclerosis. Neurol Clin 2005; 23:1–15.
5. Larocca NG. Impact of walking impairment in multiple sclerosis: perspectives of patients and care partners. Patient 2011;4:189–201.
6. Murray TJ. Multiple sclerosis: the history of a disease. New York: Demos; 2005.
7. Hobart JC, Riazi A, Lamping DL, et al. Measuring the impact of MS on walking ability: the 12-item MS Walking Scale (MSWS-12). Neurology 2003;60:31–6.
8. Van Asch P. Impact of mobility impairment in multiple sclerosis 2 – Patients' perspectives. Eur Neurol Rev 2011;6:115–20.
9. Pearson OR, Busse ME, Van Deursen RW, et al. Quantification of walking mobility in neurological disorders. QJM 2004;97:463–75.
10. Sosnoff JJ, Gappmaier E, Frame A, et al. Influence of spasticity on mobility and balance in persons with multiple sclerosis. J Neurol Phys Ther 2011;35: 129–32.
11. Huisinga JM, Filipi ML, Schmid KK, et al. Is there a relationship between fatigue questionnaires and gait mechanisms in persons with multiple sclerosis? Arch Phys Med Rehabil 2011;92:1594–601.
12. Motl RW, Sandroff BM, Suh Y, et al. Energy cost of walking and its association with gait parameters, daily activity, and fatigue in persons with mild multiple sclerosis. Neurorehabil Neural Repair 2012;26:1015–21.
13. Martin CL, Phillips BA, Kilpatrick TJ, et al. Gait and balance impairment in early multiple sclerosis in the absence of clinical disability. Mult Scler 2006;12:620–8.
14. Saunders JB, Inman VT, Eberthart HD. The major determinants in normal and pathological gait. J Bone Joint Surg Am 1953;35:543–58.

15. Orendurff MS, Segal AD, Klute GK, et al. The effect of walking speed on center of mass displacement. J Rehabil Res Dev 2004;41:829–34.
16. Motl RW, Sandroff BM, Sosnoff JJ. Commercially available accelerometry as an ecologically valid measure of ambulation in persons with multiple sclerosis. Expert Rev Neurother 2012;12:1079–88.
17. Iezzoni LI. When walking fails. Mobility problems of adults with chronic conditions. Berkeley (CA): University of California Press; 2003.
18. Heesen C, Böhm J, Reich C, et al. Patient perception of bodily functions in multiple sclerosis: gait and visual function are the most valuable. Mult Scler 2008;14:988–91.
19. Motl RW, Snook EM, McAuley E, et al. Demographic correlates of physical activity in individuals with multiple sclerosis. Disabil Rehabil 2007;29:1301–4.
20. Gijbels D, Alders G, Van Hoof E, et al. Predicting habitual walking performance in multiple sclerosis: relevance of capacity and self-report measures. Mult Scler 2010;16:618–26.
21. Goldman MD, Motl RW, Rudick RA. Possible clinical outcome measures for clinical trials in patients with multiple sclerosis. Ther Adv Neurol Disord 2010;3(4): 229–39.
22. Kurtzke JF. Rating neurologic impairment in multiple sclerosis: an expanded disability status scale (EDSS). Neurology 1983;33(11):1444–52.
23. Fischer JS, Rudick RA, Cutter GR, et al. The Multiple Sclerosis Functional Composite measure (MFSC): an integrated approach to MS clinical outcome assessment. National MS Society Clinical Outcomes Assessment Task Force. Mult Scler 1999;5:244–50.
24. Confavreux C, Vukusic S. Natural history of multiple sclerosis. Brain 2006;129: 606–16.
25. Confavreux C, Vukusic S, Adeline P. Early clinical predictors and progression of irreversible disability in multiple sclerosis: an amnesic process. Brain 2003;126: 770–82.
26. Confavreux C, Vukusic S, Moreau T, et al. Relapses and progression of disability in multiple sclerosis. N Engl J Med 2000;343:1430–8.
27. Schwid SR, Goodman AD, McDermott MP, et al. Quantitative functional measures in MS: what is reliable change? Neurology 2002;58:1294–6.
28. Kieseier BC, Pozzilli C. Assessing walking disability in multiple sclerosis. Mult Scler 2012;18:914–24.
29. Phan-Ba R, Pace A, Calay P, et al. Comparison of the timed 25-foot and the 100-meter walk as performance measures in multiple sclerosis. Neurorehabil Neural Repair 2011;25:672–9.
30. Goldman MD, Marrie RA, Cohen JA. Evaluation of the six-minute walk in multiple sclerosis subjects and healthy controls. Mult Scler 2008;14:383–90.
31. Heffernan KS, Ranadive S, Weikert M, et al. Pulse pressure is associated with walking impairment in multiple sclerosis. J Neurol Sci 2011;309:105–9.
32. Motl RW, Suh Y, Balantrapu S, et al. Evidence for the different physiological significance of the 6- and 2-minute walk tests in multiple sclerosis. BMC Neurol 2012;12:6.
33. Motl RW, Weikert M, Suh Y, et al. Accuracy of the Actibelt(®) accelerometer for measuring walking speed in a controlled environment among persons with multiple sclerosis. Gait Posture 2012;35:192–6.
34. Givon U, Zeilig G, Achiron A. Gait analysis in multiple sclerosis: characterization of temporal-spatial parameters using GAITRite functional ambulation system. Gait Posture 2009;29:138–42.

35. Sosnoff JJ, Boes MK, Sandroff BM, et al. Walking and thinking in persons with multiple sclerosis who vary in disability. Arch Phys Med Rehabil 2011;92: 2028–33.
36. Sosnoff JJ, Sandroff B, Motl RW. Quantifying gait abnormalities in persons with multiple sclerosis with minimal disability. Gait Posture 2012;36:154–6.
37. Sosnoff JJ, Weikert M, Dlugonski D, et al. Quantifying gait impairment in multiple sclerosis using GAITRite™ technology. Gait Posture 2011;34:145–7.
38. Pilutti LA, Dlugonski D, Sandroff BM, et al. Further validation of Multiple Sclerosis Walking Scale-12 scores based on spatiotemporal gait parameters. Arch Phys Med Rehabil, in press.
39. Waters S, Mulroy S. The energy expenditure of normal and pathological gait. Gait Posture 1999;9:207–31.
40. Motl RW, Dlugonski D, Weikert M, et al. Multiple sclerosis walking scale-12 and oxygen cost of walking. Gait Posture 2010;31:506–10.
41. Motl RW, Snook EM, Agiovlasitit S, et al. Calibration of accelerometer output for ambulatory adults with multiple sclerosis. Arch Phys Med Rehabil 2009;90: 1778–84.
42. Motl RW, Suh Y, Dlugonski D, et al. Oxygen cost of treadmill and over-ground walking in mildly disabled persons with multiple sclerosis. Neurol Sci 2011;32: 255–62.
43. Olgiati R, Jacquet J, Di Prampero PE. Energy cost of walking and exertional dyspnea in multiple sclerosis. Am Rev Respir Dis 1986;134:1005–10.
44. Sandroff BM, Motl RW. Comparison of ActiGraph activity monitors in persons with multiple sclerosis and controls. Disabil Rehabil, in press.
45. Sosnoff JJ, Goldman MS, Motl RW. Real-life walking impairment in multiple sclerosis: preliminary comparison of four methods for processing accelerometry data. Mult Scler 2010;16:868–77.
46. Weikert M, Suh Y, Lane A, et al. Accelerometry is associated with walking mobility, not physical activity, in persons with multiple sclerosis. Med Eng Phys 2012;34: 590–7.
47. Yogev-Seligmann G, Hausdorff JM, Giladi N. The role of executive function and attention in gait. Mov Disord 2007;23:329–42.
48. Benedict RH, Holtzer R, Motl RW, et al. Upper and lower extremity motor function and cognitive impairment in multiple sclerosis. J Int Neuropsychol Soc 2011;13: 1–11.
49. Hamilton F, Rochester L, Paul L, et al. Walking and talking: an investigation of cognitive-motor dual tasking in multiple sclerosis. Mult Scler 2009;15:1215–27.
50. Kalron A, Dvir Z, Achiron A. Walking while talking—difficulties incurred during the initial stages of multiple sclerosis disease process. Gait Posture 2010;32:332–5.
51. Hersch C, Rae-Grant A. Extended-release dalfampridine in the management of multiple-sclerosis-related walking impairment. Ther Adv Neurol Disord 2012;5: 199–204.
52. Blight AR. Treatment of walking impairment in multiple sclerosis with dalfampridine. Ther Adv Neurol Disord 2011;4:99–109.
53. Goodman AD, Brown TR, Krupp LB, et al. Sustained-release oral fampridine in multiple sclerosis: a randomised, double-blind, controlled trial. Lancet 2009; 373:732–8.
54. Goodman AD, Brown TR, Edwards KR, et al. A phase 3 trial of extended release oral dalfampridine in multiple sclerosis. Ann Neurol 2010;68:494–502.
55. Shakespeare DT, Boggild M, Young C. Anti-spasticity agents for multiple sclerosis. Cochrane Database Syst Rev 2003;(4):CD001332.

56. Motl RW. Physical activity and irreversible disability in multiple sclerosis. Exerc Sport Sci Rev 2010;38:186–91.

57. Motl RW, Goldman MD, Benedict RH. Walking impairment in patients with multiple sclerosis: exercise training as a treatment option? Neuropsychiatr Dis Treat 2010; 6:767–74.

58. Motl RW, Pilutti LA. The benefits of exercise training in multiple sclerosis. Nat Rev Neurol 2012;8:487–97.

59. Snook EM, Motl RW. Effect of exercise training on walking mobility in multiple sclerosis: a meta-analysis. Neurorehabil Neural Repair 2009;23:108–16.

60. Motl RW, Smith DC, Elliott J, et al. Combined training improves walking mobility in persons with significant disability from multiple sclerosis: a pilot study. J Neurol Phys Ther 2012;36:32–7.

61. Beer S, Aschbacher B, Manoglou D, et al. Robot-assisted gait training in multiple sclerosis: a pilot randomized trial. Mult Scler 2008;14:231–6.

62. Geisser B, Beres-Jones J, Budovitch A, et al. Locomotor training using body weight support on a treadmill improves mobility in persons with multiple sclerosis: a pilot study. Mult Scler 2007;13:224–31.

63. Lo AC, Triche EW. Improving gait in multiple sclerosis using robot-assisted, body weight supported treadmill training. Neurorehabil Neural Repair 2008;22:661–71.

64. Pilutti LA, Lelli DA, Paulseth JE, et al. Effects of 12 weeks of supported treadmill training on functional ability and quality of life in progressive multiple sclerosis: a pilot study. Arch Phys Med Rehabil 2011;92:31–6.

65. Kelleher KJ, Spence W, Solomonidis S, et al. Ambulatory rehabilitation in multiple sclerosis. Disabil Rehabil 2009;31:1625–32.

66. Wiles CM. Physiotherapy and related activities in multiple sclerosis. Mult Scler 2008;14:863–71.

67. Vaney C, Gattlen B, Lugon-Moulin V, et al. Robotic-assisted step training (Lokomat) not superior to equal intensity of over-ground rehabilitation in patients with multiple sclerosis. Neurorehabil Neural Repair 2012;26(3):212–21.

68. Prakash RS, Snook EM, Erickson KI, et al. Cardiorespiratory fitness: a predictor of cortical plasticity in multiple sclerosis. Neuroimage 2007;34:1238–44.

69. Prakash RS, Snook EM, Motl RW, et al. Aerobic fitness is associated with gray matter volume and white matter integrity in multiple sclerosis. Brain Res 2010; 1341:41–51.

70. Motl RW, Sandroff BM, Benedict RH. Cognitive dysfunction and multiple sclerosis: developing a rationale for considering the efficacy of exercise training. Mult Scler 2011;17:1034–40.

71. Bartrés-Faz D, Arenaza-Urquijo EM. Structural and functional imaging correlates of cognitive and brain reserve hypotheses in healthy and pathological aging. Brain Topogr 2011;24:340–57.

72. Colcombe SJ, Kramer AF, McAuley E, et al. Neurocognitive aging and cardiovascular fitness: recent findings and future directions. J Mol Neurosci 2004;24:9–14.

Measurement and Treatment of Imbalance and Fall Risk in Multiple Sclerosis Using the International Classification of Functioning, Disability and Health Model

Michelle H. Cameron, MD, PT[a],*, Ylva E. Nilsagård, PT, PhD[b,c]

KEYWORDS

- Multiple sclerosis • Accidental falls • Gait • Walking • Postural balance

KEY POINTS

- Impaired balance and walking are common in people with multiple sclerosis (MS).
- The International Classification of Functioning, Disability and Health provides an ideal framework for organizing the examination and assessment of imbalance, fall risk, and impaired walking in people with MS.
- Balance and fall measures make important contributions in directing therapeutic interventions and potentially for assessing the effectiveness of both disease-modifying and symptomatic interventions.

INTRODUCTION

Multiple sclerosis (MS) is the most common nontraumatic neurologic disease of young adults. Worldwide, approximately 2.5 million people are diagnosed with MS.[1] MS is characterized by variable neurologic symptoms, disease activity, and progression of functional limitations over time. Many people with MS (PwMS) report that ambulation is affected by their disease. PwMS walk more slowly than healthy controls and their balance is also impaired compared with healthy controls. PwMS also fall frequently. Even before walking is slowed, PwMS have balance impairments, which can be detected by clinical and instrumented measures.[2] The focus of this article is the measurement and treatment of imbalance and fall risk in PwMS.

[a] Department of Neurology, Oregon Health and Science University, 3181 Southwest Sam Jackson Park Road, L226 Portland, OR 97239, USA; [b] Centre for Health Care Sciences, Örebro County Council, P.O Box 1324, Örebro SE-701 13, Sweden; [c] School of Health and Medical Sciences, Örebro University, Örebro, SE-701 85, Sweden
* Corresponding author.
E-mail address: cameromi@ohsu.edu

Phys Med Rehabil Clin N Am 24 (2013) 337–354
http://dx.doi.org/10.1016/j.pmr.2012.11.009
1047-9651/13/$ – see front matter © 2013 Elsevier Inc. All rights reserved.

Balance measures can identify individuals with impaired balance and at increased risk for falls. Some measures also identify specific impairments of body function and structure contributing to imbalance and can assess the impact of imbalance and falls on a person's level of activity and ability to participate in usual activities. High-quality (precise, reliable, and valid) measures of imbalance and fall risk are essential for identifying who may benefit from interventions to improve balance and reduce fall risk, and for selecting the most appropriate interventions. In addition, balance and fall measures may overcome some of the limitations of tools currently used to assess the effectiveness of disease-modifying and symptomatic interventions, as discussed in detail later in this article.

Imbalance, or reduced postural control, is present and detectable in most PwMS. Imbalance can be the initial symptom of MS[3] and has been found even in those with minimal changes on clinical examination.[4–7] Balance impairment also generally persists and becomes more pronounced as MS progresses.[8–10] Studies have found consistent differences in balance control between PwMS and healthy individuals.[11–13] PwMS have 3 related balance control abnormalities. First, they have decreased ability to maintain position when attempting to stand still[5,6,9,10,14–16]; second, they have limited and slowed movement toward their limits of stability when attempting to lean or reach[7,9,17,18]; and third, they have delayed automatic postural responses when displaced or perturbed.[8,13,19,20] In quiet stance, PwMS sway more than healthy controls and this postural sway increases even more than in controls with eyes closed and is greater in those with more impairment (higher Expanded Disability Status Scale [EDSS] scores) and in those with progressive MS.[21] When initiating a step to start to walk, or when reaching, PwMS move less far and less quickly than healthy controls. Furthermore, PwMS have delayed automatic postural responses when the support surface they are standing on moves.

Imbalance affects quality of life and the performance of almost all daily activities. Imbalance not only affects walking but can also cause falls or near falls, both of which are common in PwMS,[22–27] and falls can cause injury[28] and fear of falling.[29–31] Up to 63% of randomly selected samples of PwMS report having fallen at least once over the past 1 to 12 months, and many fall more often.[22–27,29] Falls can occur early in the course of MS,[32] although the risk seems to increase with increasing level of disability[23,24,26,27] as long as the person is ambulatory (although falls may also occur during transfers in nonambulatory PwMS). Falls in PwMS are associated with injuries, most commonly fractures.[31] In a Danish cohort of more than 11,000 PwMS, there were 22.8 fractures per 1000 person-years.[33] Hip fractures were the most common followed by fractures of the radius/ulna, tibia, and femur. In middle-aged and older PwMS, an injurious fall is associated with increased fear of falling[31] and activity curtailment.[31] Whether or not a PwMS has fallen in the past 6 months, more than 70% report being concerned about falling.[29] Fear of falling and the consequent inactivity can perpetuate a pattern of deconditioning, further balance impairment, and increased fall risk, as well as accelerated bone loss and an increased risk for fall-related fractures. Although near falls rarely result in injury and may prompt a PwMS to take steps to prevent future falls, near falls also likely increase fear of falling and reduce activity, self-esteem, and self-confidence. Poor postural control can also increase the energy demand of walking[34] and other daily activities and thus increase fatigue and limit a person's activity.

The high prevalence of imbalance and its significant consequences in PwMS makes imbalance important to recognize, quantify, and treat. Certain balance measures may also be able to guide intervention by determining the mechanisms contributing to imbalance. Various mechanisms have been proposed to underlie imbalance and falls in MS, including slowed somatosensory conduction,[8,13,19,35,36] impaired central integration,[8,13,19,35,36] weakness,[24] and spasticity.[26,37,38] In interviews, PwMS also report that impairments of attention, muscular endurance, gait pattern, vision, and proprioception, as well as heat sensitivity and fatigue, cause them to fall.[39] Being able to identify, quantify, and understand the contributors to imbalance and increased fall risk in PwMS is essential for optimizing treatment. In this article, the roles and advantages of balance and fall measures in PwMS are discussed, specific balance and fall measures at different levels of the International Classification of Functioning, Disability and Health (ICF) model are identified, and the multidimensionality of falls is shown using the ICF model.[40]

Assessment of Imbalance and Fall Risk Using the ICF Model

We recommend using the ICF model to structure the assessment of imbalance and fall risk in PwMS. The ICF model is also recommended for structuring the assessment of walking limitations in PwMS and for the assessment of imbalance, fall risk, and walking limitations in people with other central nervous system (CNS) disorders such as Parkinson disease or Alzheimer disease. This model was developed by the World Health Organization to provide a standardized language and structure for describing health and health-related conditions.[40] According to the ICF model, health is the result of a complex interaction between functioning, disability, and contextual factors. Functioning and disability are made up of 3 components: body function and structure, activities, and participation. Contextual factors include environmental and personal factors (**Fig. 1**). The ICF model facilitates clear and complete communication among health care providers concerning complex health problems. Imbalance, falls, and walking limitations in people with CNS disorders are complex health problems that can affect performance of a wide range of activities and participation in roles at home, at work, and in the community and that generally involve several professions to achieve optimal solutions. The ICF model can help identify possible causes, contributors, and ameliorators of imbalance, falls, and walking problems and may suggest solutions that can be provided by various health care team members to address 1 or more components of the model.

Roles and advantages of balance and fall measures in MS

Although balance and fall measures focus only on certain specific consequences of MS and do not provide information about the status or changes in processes underlying MS, including inflammation, demyelination, and neurodegeneration, these measures are suited to identifying PwMS with imbalance and at risk for falls and for

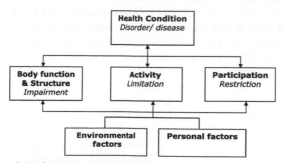

Fig. 1. The ICF model of health and health-related conditions: a complex interaction between functioning, disability and contextual factors.

directing interventions to address these problems. In addition, in PwMS, particularly those with progressive MS, these measures may represent useful adjunctive tools for assessing disease progression and the impact of other interventions, because they overcome some of the limitations of current measurement tools, including magnetic resonance imaging (MRI), relapse rate, EDSS,[41] and MS Functional Composite (MSFC)[42] scale.

MRI is an excellent tool for assisting in the diagnosis of MS and can be used to assess disease progression and activity. Most PwMS have characteristic lesions on brain MRI, and MS is almost uniquely associated with spinal cord lesions appreciable on MRI. During the relapsing phase of the disease, disease activity is reflected by an increase in the number, size, and overall volume of lesions on MRI and the presence of gadolinium-enhancing lesions. However, MRI is expensive and time-consuming, lesions generally evolve slowly over time, there is poor correlation between MRI lesion volume and location with physical abilities, and MRI is relatively insensitive to changes associated with progressive MS. The EDSS, a measure of neurologic function in 8 functional systems (visual, brainstem, pyramidal, cerebellar, sensory, bowel and bladder, cerebral, and other) in which a significant part of the scoring range is based on ambulation status, can be used to quantify MS progression and response to treatment and captures some aspects of body structure and function and some aspects of activity. However, it has poor intrarater and interrater reliability,[43,44] does not assess other aspects of activity or any aspects of participation, and has limited precision, being a 20-point scale (0–10 including half-points). The MSFC, a 3-part multidimensional standardized composite clinical measure designed for use in clinical trials in MS,[42] includes a simple timed measure of ambulation (the timed 7.62-m [25-ft] walk), a measure of upper extremity function (the 9-hole peg test), and a measure of cognitive function (the Paced Auditory Serial Addition Test [PASAT]). Although the MSFC may be more responsive to change than the EDSS, captures a range of activities, and correlates with MRI changes, it is limited by practice effects and floor and ceiling effects and does not assess participation or contextual factors.

In contrast to traditional MS measures, balance and fall measures can be inexpensive and quick, may detect change over a short period, are direct measures of physical abilities, and may also be more sensitive to gradual changes occurring in the absence of relapses, which can be particularly helpful in people with progressive MS. Balance and fall measures have also been found to correlate with EDSS scores[23,27,45] and, although focused on lower extremity function, may provide more information than traditional measures do about activities and about the impact of activity limitations on participation; they can also predict who is at increased risk for falls.

Balance and fall measures at different levels of the ICF

A wide range of measures are available to assess balance and falls in PwMS. These measures include simple patient-completed questionnaires and a range of clinical tests and test batteries, as well as technologically advanced instrumented measures. Early in the course of MS, when imbalance can be subtle, patients may report imbalance despite current clinical measures not being sensitive enough to detect problems. In this circumstance, instrumented measures can be helpful because they often detect objective balance control deficits. Measure selection depends on the purpose of the measurement and the technical, personnel, and time resources available. The measures discussed in this article are those most often reported being used in published articles indexed in PubMed to February 2012 using the search strategy: "postural balance" OR "accidental falls" AND "multiple sclerosis," and other measures that may provide substantial advantages over these commonly used measures.

BODY FUNCTION AND STRUCTURE

Impairments in body function and structure, such as reduced muscle strength, altered muscle tone and coordination, altered gait pattern, reduced joint mobility, impaired sensation, impaired vision, fatigue, and impaired attention and cognitive function, are common in PwMS and may contribute to fall risk individually or in combination. Many measures are available to assess body function and structure, including posturography, MRI, the EDSS, and neurologic examination.

Muscle strength is required for body movement, and lower extremity muscle strength is required for standing and walking. Reduced lower extremity strength is associated with an increased risk of falling in women with MS.[24] Strong abdominal and back muscles are also needed to stabilize the trunk when moving the extremities while walking. Weak proximal muscles can contribute to reduced lower extremity movement during the swing phase of gait and reduced stability during stance phase and can also impair knee stabilization during stance, leading to hyperextension. Weak ankle dorsiflexors, or increased ankle plantarflexor or hip adductor tone, may also cause tripping and stumbling. Upper extremity spasticity may also increase fall risk for people who use hand-held assistive devices for mobility. Muscle strength and tone can be tested using manual resistance of the tester, functional tests (eg, getting up from a chair), and with various devices (eg, spring or isokinetic dynamometers). Spasticity should be assessed both at rest and during functional activities because tone may change with position and activity. The modified Ashworth scale is commonly used to quantify spasticity at rest.[46] Poor coordination, often as a result of cerebellar ataxia, may also contribute to an altered gait pattern, gait instability, and falls.

Altered gait pattern and reduced joint mobility may be the result of reduced strength, spasticity,[38] ataxia, or sensory (including proprioceptive) loss. Gait pattern changes common in PwMS include reduced stride length,[7,47] prolonged double limb support time,[7,47] abnormal muscle recruitment,[47] and gait initiation,[18] as well as reduced maximum hip and knee extension and ankle plantar flexion range of motion.[48] Gait pattern can be analyzed visually by observational gait analysis, or using an instrumented walkway.[49] Instrumented walkways can measure various spatiotemporal parameters of gait and have shown that specific gait patterns are associated with EDSS functional scores.[50] More sophisticated motion analysis systems, as provided in a gait laboratory or using gyroscopes and accelerometers worn by the patient, may provide additional useful information about gait kinetics and kinematics for research but are not available routinely in clinical practice.

Impaired touch and position sensation in the lower extremities is also associated with impaired postural control[10,13] in PwMS and increases the risk for falls. Proprioception can be quickly assessed by estimating or matching the position of the great toe. Somatosensory-evoked potential testing can be used to more precisely quantify and localize somatosensory conduction abnormalities in the CNS. Although use of another reliable sensory input, usually vision, can compensate for impaired lower limb proprioceptive function to facilitate balance,[10] in PwMS, visual dysfunction caused by optic neuritis (which can cause blurred vision and blind spots), and internuclear ophthalmoplegia or other oculomotor dysfunction (which can cause diplopia), often limit the use of visual substitution to improve balance. Visual impairment alone increases the risk for falls and further increases fall risk when combined with loss of proprioception. Visual acuity and oculomotor function are both evaluated as part of the EDSS and in the typical neurologic examination.

Fatigue can contribute to fall risk in PwMS by exacerbating other symptoms. In a systematic review of measurement properties of self-report fatigue questionnaires validated in individuals with a neurologic diagnosis, the Fatigue Scale for Motor and Cognitive (FSMC) functions and the Unidimensional Fatigue Impact Scale (U-FIS) were recommended for PwMS.[51] The FSMC contains 10 cognitive and 10 motor dimensions rating fatigue in general using a 5-point Likert scale, giving a score range between 20 and 100.[52] The U-FIS captures the impact of fatigue in the last week using 22 items covering one dimension rated by a 4-point Likert scale with a score ranging from 0 to 66.[53,54] Other reliable fatigue scales developed for PwMS are the Modified Fatigue Impact Scale (MFIS) and the Fatigue Severity Scale (FSS).[55] The MFIS is an MS-specific 21-item questionnaire evaluating the impact of fatigue on cognitive, physical, and psychosocial functioning. The MFIS is based on items derived from interviews with PwMS about how fatigue affects their lives. Scores on the MFIS range from 0 to 84, with lower scores indicating less fatigue. There is no published cutoff score for defining fatigue with the MFIS. The FSS is a 9-item questionnaire, which asks individuals to rate the degree to which fatigue affects their lives. Scores on the FSS range from 1 to 7, with lower scores indicating less fatigue. A cutoff score of greater than or equal to 5 on the FSS has been suggested to discriminate between fatigued and nonfatigued individuals.[56] These fatigue measures are both validated and commonly used in drug and rehabilitation treatment trials in MS.[57,58]

Impaired attention and cognitive function can also affect postural control, as shown by the worsening of postural control and gait impairment during dual task performance in PwMS.[3,59–61] Gait slows and other spatiotemporal parameters of gait worsen more in PwMS than in healthy controls when a cognitive task is performed while walking.[62] These changes are more pronounced in those with severe (EDSS 6.0–6.5) and moderate disability (EDSS 4.0–5.5) than in those with mild disability (EDSS 2.0–3.5). Postural control for other tasks also declines during dual task conditions in PwMS, with the greatest declines in those with higher EDSS scores.[61] Attention and processing speed can be assessed by several tests, including the PASAT, which is a component of the MSFC. The Symbol Digit Modalities Test (SDMT, oral form) is another widely used test of attention and processing speed. Compared with the PASAT, the SDMT is less time-consuming, requires less equipment, and has good psychometric properties.[63] The SDMT is recommended for use when personnel with neuropsychological training are lacking.[64]

Computerized dynamic posturography (CDP) is the balance measurement tool most commonly used in published research. CDP uses a motorized platform and visual surround to assess static and dynamic balance directly. CDP equipment has the advantage of providing precise information about standing balance, postural sway and responses to perturbations of visual, proprioceptive, and vestibular input.[11] However, use of CDP is limited by the expense of the equipment (~$100,000 US) as well as the significant dedicated space requirements, specialized software products, and advanced training needs. These resource requirements have generally limited the use of CDP to research or specialty clinical settings. CDP has been used extensively to study postural control in MS as well as in many other populations and many control and comparison data are available. Recently, less expensive (~$15,000 US) small wearable devices with gyroscopes and inertial sensors that precisely monitor movement to assess dynamic balance during walking have become commercially available. These newer devices also provide detailed information about postural control and have been shown to detect postural control deficits in PwMS whose walking is not slow.[2] Use of these devices is limited by the lack of standard testing protocols and the absence of established reliability and validity in specific populations. Once standard testing protocols are developed and reliability and validity are established, it is likely that these wearable devices will contribute significantly to the study of postural control as well as walking in PwMS and people with other CNS disorders.

In addition to the specific measures of body function and structure discussed earlier, a clinical test battery, the Postural Physiologic Assessment (PPA), which involves simple tests of vision, peripheral sensation, muscle force, reaction time, and postural sway, has been developed to predict fall risk in elderly individuals.[65] This battery has proven validity in older adults, and its validity in PwMS is currently being studied. For the PPA, postural sway in standing is assessed with the sway meter, a simple device with a pen attached to a horizontal bar extending from a belt worn around the pelvis (**Fig. 2**). The PPA uses other portable inexpensive low-tech equipment for other components of testing, and a computer program is available to compare individual data with normative data.

ACTIVITY

Most clinically administered balance tests focus on the ability to maintain balance during specific activities. The EDSS, which focuses on information about body function and structure, also assesses aspects of walking activity, including the distance a person can walk and the amount of assistance they need to walk. The MSFC is entirely a measure of activity and measures walking speed, upper extremity function, and cognition. The Timed Up and Go test (TUG), the Berg Balance Scale (BBS), the Dynamic Gait Index (DGI) and, the Functional Reach Test (FRT) are all measures of activity associated with balance commonly used in PwMS. These tools measure capacity (ie, what a person can do), but not performance (ie, what they do).

The TUG was developed to test basic mobility skills in frail elderly people and is the clinical test of balance most commonly used in published studies in PwMS. To perform the TUG, the individual stands up from sitting in a chair, walks 3 m, turns around, walks back to the chair, and sits back down. The TUG score is the time in seconds taken to perform this task.[66] The TUG is quick and easy to administer and has been widely used in several populations, including PwMS. The TUG can also be performed easily in many settings, including most homes and clinics, and its reliability

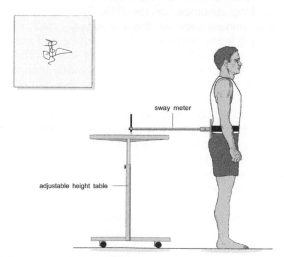

Fig. 2. The sway meter in the physiologic profile assessment. (*Courtesy of* Stephen Lord, PhD, University of New South Wales, Sydney, Australia.)

is established.[67,68] The TUG has good face validity for predicting who will fall, because falls in PwMS often occur during transfers, walking, and turning.[25,39] However, when performed alone, the TUG was found to discriminate poorly between fallers and non-fallers with MS,[69] although when performed together with a cognitive task (backward counting by 3s), it performed well, correctly identifying 73% of the fallers (positive predictive value) using a cutoff score of 13.6 seconds or more (sensitivity 48%; specificity 73%).[26] Normative values have been published for healthy people aged 20 to 29 years (5.31 ± 0.25 seconds)[70] and 70 to 79 years (8–8.54 seconds),[66,70–72] but reference values are lacking for PwMS.

The BBS[73] was developed to measure balance in older adults and is used almost as frequently as the TUG to assess balance performance in PwMS. The BBS addresses 2 dimensions of balance: the ability to maintain upright posture and the ability to make appropriate adjustments for voluntary movement. Narrowing the base of support, asking individuals to lean toward the edges of the base of support and altering sensory input manipulate the difficulty of the test. The BBS takes 15 to 20 minutes to administer and has established reliability in PwMS.[68,74] Advantages of the BBS are that several of the tasks used in the test are related to daily activities and that it tests the ability to maintain balance without visual input and with a narrow base of support, providing information that may help direct therapy. Various BBS cutoff scores can discriminate between fallers (≥1 fall the past 3 months) and nonfallers with MS. A cutoff score of 55 or less (close to the maximum score of 56) predicted falls in the following 3 months with high sensitivity (94%) but limited specificity (32%).[26] Alternatively, a cutoff score of more than 44 was 90% specific but only 40% sensitive in its association with falls in the previous month.[69] A cutoff score with both high sensitivity and high specificity for identifying fallers has not been determined for this scale. Ceiling and floor effects in PwMS also limit the usefulness of this scale and the test cannot assess performance in those who are not able to stand.

The DGI was developed to assess the likelihood of falling in older adults. The DGI assesses performance on 8 walking tasks, including changing gait speed, turning, stepping over obstacles, stair walking, and walking with head movements. The maximum score, which indicates better performance, is 24. This 15-minute to 20-minute test provides richer information about walking activities required for daily life than gait speed, maximum walking distance, or the TUG. The DGI has been validated in PwMS.[69,75] It can discriminate between those reporting a fall in the past month and those reporting not falling in the past month,[69,75] using a cutoff score of more than 12 (sensitivity 45%; specificity 80%).[69] The optimal cutoff score for the DGI for predicting future falls in PwMS needs to be established. The total walking distance required by the DGI also limits its use for PwMS with an EDSS of 6.0 or less, and the last item requires access to stairs.

The FRT was developed as a quick screen for balance problems in older adults. The FRT measures maximal forward reach with a fixed base of support with 1 arm raised to 90°.[76] Normative values have been published for healthy people,[76] and the test has been found to discriminate between PwMS diagnosed recently[7] or many years ago (median 6.5 years)[17] and healthy controls. This test requires only a wall to stand next to and a ruler and is quickly administered, but it can be difficult to control for trunk rotation during the reach.

In addition to these tests, the Four Square Step Test (FSST) was recently developed as a quick and simple test to predict fall risk in older adults[77] and has also been used in research and clinical practice with PwMS. The FSST involves the person stepping in sequence forward, sideways, backward, and sideways first clockwise and then counterclockwise over canes placed in a cross formation. This test is quick and easy to administer and mimics daily activities, including basic weight shifting and lifting the foot over lower obstacles such as carpets and thresholds, and may be a good test for detecting trips, which are a common cause of falls in PwMS.[25] Using a cutoff of 16.9 seconds or more, in PwMS, this test has a positive predictive value of 81% for predicting who will fall in the following 3 months.[26]

The Balance Evaluation Systems Test (BESTest) is a new clinical test battery initially developed to assess balance control in people with Parkinson disease.[78] The BESTest assesses the following 6 systems contributing to postural control: biomechanical constraints, stability limits/verticality, anticipatory postural adjustments, postural responses, sensory orientation, and stability in gait. This test is a measure of activity and includes tasks such as maintaining balance while standing on different surfaces, walking, transferring, reaching, in-place responses, and compensatory stepping reactions. The BESTest is now being validated in PwMS. A shorter version of the BESTest, the miniBESTest, which takes 15 to 20 minutes rather than 30 to 40 minutes, is also available.[79] The comprehensiveness of the BESTest and its potential to direct intervention give this test considerable potential for clinical and research applications in PwMS.

Timed walk tests may also provide information about balance and postural control in PwMS but are beyond the scope of this article. The 10-m walk test[67] and the timed 7.62-m (25-ft) walk[80] are both reliable measures of walking speed in PwMS, and the modified 6-minute walk test is a reliable and valid measure of walking endurance in PwMS. The 6-minute walk test has been found to discriminate between EDSS subgroups.[81,82]

PARTICIPATION

Clear differentiation between activity and participation is challenging and not always strived for. Limitations in activities may or may not restrict participation, depending on environmental and personal factors, such as using an assistive device or other coping or compensatory strategies. Nonetheless, restrictions in participation, particularly restrictions in recreation and leisure participation,[83] are common in PwMS. In addition, PwMS are often restricted in aspects of participation such as moving around, acquiring goods and services, community life, and community mobility.[84] Measures of community integration have been suggested to capture participation as well as individual and contextual factors, and physical, social, and psychological dimensions.[85] Most measures of participation are generic rather than disease-specific, and few studies of imbalance and falls in PwMS have used these measures.

The Impact on Participation and Autonomy Questionnaire (IPAQ) assesses the subjectively perceived impact of chronic disability on autonomy and participation.[86] The IPAQ includes 5 domains: social relations, autonomy in self-care, mobility and leisure, family role, work and educational opportunities, and a composite overall perceived participation. The IPAQ is valid and reliable in people with chronic disorders, including neurologic disorders.[86] To our knowledge, the validity and reliability of the IPAQ in PwMS has not been evaluated.

The Community Integration Questionnaire (CIQ) was originally developed as a measure of community integration for people with traumatic brain injury and consists of 15 items relevant to the domains of home integration, social integration, and productive activities.[87] The CIQ has been validated for use with populations with spinal cord injury (SCI)[88] and has been used in studies in PwMS.[89] The CIQ has also been found to be a valid measure of participation in a heterogeneous sample of adults with physical disability, with some small modifications to the scoring system to optimize its use.[90] The CIQ is also easily administered.[85]

The Craig Handicap Assessment and Reporting Technique (CHART) was designed to measure the level of handicap in community-living people with SCI.[91] The CHART collects information on the degree to which the respondent fulfills the roles typically expected from people without disabilities. The CHART is a 32-item questionnaire, and the questions can be answered in a quantifiable way (eg, hours of assistance). There is also a 19-question short form of the CHART. Each dimension is scored on a 0 to 100 scale. Norms and profiles of CHART scores for many populations have been published, and the CHART has shown reliability in PwMS.

The MS Impact Profile (MSIP) is an MS-specific ICF-based outcome measure designed to assess 4 components of the ICF, one being participation in life situations.[92] The impact is measured by 5 questions covering environmental obstacles that complicate mobility, personal care, relationships, employment, or community, recreation, and leisure. A 5-graded response scale ranges from 0 (no) to 4 (yes, as a consequence ... is (nearly) impossible). The MSIP is reliable and valid in PwMS[92,93] and provides information not only about disability but also about the perception of disability, which can be important for tailoring interventions to the individual.

PERSONAL FACTORS

Personal factors related to balance and falls can be measured with self-report questionnaires about balance confidence and the individual's perception of their abilities or limitations. The Activities-specific Balance Confidence Scale (ABC) and the Dizziness Handicap Inventory (DHI) are balance self-rating scales used frequently in MS research to assess personal factors related to balance and falls.

The ABC[94] is a 16-item questionnaire developed to measure balance confidence in older adults. ABC scores range from 0 (no confidence) to 100 (completely confident). The ABC addresses indoor and outdoor activities and targets a person's strength (confidence) rather than weakness (fear). However, it is culturally specific, requiring people to assess their confidence performing activities that they may perform rarely or never, such as walking on icy sidewalks and stepping onto or off an escalator. It has been found to be valid[69,95] and reliable in PwMS.[74] The ABC was reported to be 65% sensitive and 77% specific for discriminating between PwMS who have or have not fallen in the past month[69] and to discriminate between multiple fallers and nonfallers as well as between users and nonusers of assistive walking devices.[95]

The DHI is a 25-item questionnaire developed to measure the self-perceived negative consequences of vestibular system disease.[96] The items assess the functional, emotional, and physical effects of dizziness and unsteadiness. The DHI has been found to be valid[69] and reliable[74] in PwMS. The DHI provides information about emotions, such as fear of appearing intoxicated, fear of staying home alone, and feelings of embarrassment, frustration, and depression. The DHI also addresses environmental factors by asking if the problem has placed stress on relationships with family members or friends and if the person feels that they need company to leave home or walk outdoors. With a cutoff of less than 59, the DHI correctly identifies nonfallers with 74% accuracy.[69]

The Falls Efficacy Scale-International (FES-I), based on the Falls Efficacy Scale developed by Tinetti and colleagues[97] but with added questions to address the social dimension of fear of falling, is a 16-item questionnaire designed to measure perceived self-efficacy at avoiding falls during essential nonhazardous activities of daily living in community-living older adults.[98] Although the FES-I has not commonly been used in studies in PwMS, it is recommended for future studies because it was specifically designed to be used across cultures and has excellent measurement qualities in people with cognitive impairment.[99] Scores on the FES-I range from 16 to 64, with lower scores representing less fear of falling and higher confidence in performing the assessed activities.

Self-perceived walking limitations may also be affected by imbalance and can be assessed in PwMS using the MS-specific 12-item MS Walking Scale (MSWS-12).[100] Using a cutoff of 75 or more, the MSWS-12 identifies 4 of 5 nonfallers (specificity 82%).[26] It has been found valid[100–103] and reliable[100,104] in PwMS. The MSWS-12 captures more aspects of walking than traditional timed walk tests, but it cannot assess balance or fall risk in those who cannot walk.

In general, self-report questionnaires are quick to administer and may detect subtle or early imbalance that is not readily detected with other objective measures. They also can reliably detect people at low risk for falls (nonfallers). Self-report question-naires focus on the personal impact of imbalance on a person's life and function. These measures often provide information that can guide the type and amount of rehabilitation interventions needed, including addressing abilities and feelings about those abilities. However, interventions should not rely solely on subjective measures, because a person's perception of function may not accurately reflect their abilities, as supported by the finding that correlations between different self-rating scales are often higher than correlations between self-rated measures and clinical measures.[69,101,105] The reliability and validity of self-report questionnaires can be affected by inadequate insight into self-limitations, for example, when the person is asked to rate activities not performed in a long time or when they are not aware that they have made adjustments to accommodate their disability or may even be in denial of their limitations. However, cognitive dysfunction in PwMS does not seem to affect reliability or validity of self-reported measures,[106] although having personnel available to clarify the instructions can be useful.

ENVIRONMENT

PwMS have identified various environmental factors, including assistive devices, climate and weather, design and construction of public buildings, as risk factors or protective factors for falls.[39] The use of assistive devices is consistently associated with a higher risk of falls,[22,23,26] likely reflecting that assistive devices are one of the most common interventions used by people with impaired balance or who have fallen. Family members, friends, and health professionals and their attitudes can help prevent falls.[39,83] Emotional and practical support can facilitate performing activities and participation in life situations. Health care providers should recognize the importance of providing support and education not only to the patient with MS but also to signif-icant people in their lives. Climate and weather have been reported as the most signif-icant barrier to full functioning in PwMS[83] and have been identified as causing falls in PwMS.[39] PwMS report that warm ambient temperatures, caused by sunshine or other factors, exacerbate most symptoms of MS, including weakness, sensory changes, and fatigue, and that these can cause falls. Furthermore, cold or windy weather can increase spasticity and thereby also increase fall risk. There are no standardized outcome measures for environmental factors. Instead, selected variables are usually assessed using tools designed for a specific study. In this circumstance, we suggest using the ICF to assist in selection of the appropriate variables.

Using the ICF Model to Manage Imbalance and Falls in MS

Given the range and complex interactions of factors that contribute to imbalance and falls in PwMS, it is not surprising that no single measure can assess all aspects and that no single measure strongly and reliably predicts who will fall. The ICF provides an ideal framework for organizing the aspects that should be assessed in a PwMS believed to be at risk for imbalance and falls. This model is also ideal for assessing a PwMS who is having problems with walking and can guide collection of information and then selection of interventions at all levels of the ICF. **Fig. 3** shows how information from an individual case can be organized.

CLINICAL RECOMMENDATIONS AND SUMMARY

In the clinical setting, we recommend that imbalance and fall risk measures be selected based on findings from the medical provider's examination complemented by evaluation by a multidisciplinary MS specialty team. Evaluation should include the history of falls and imbalance, including factors surrounding these events, a physical examination, and a targeted combination of self-administered, clinician-administered, and instrumented measures of balance. The ICF model can help with the selection of test measures, interpretation and organization of findings, selection and administration of interventions, and assessment of change over time or in response to interventions. The ICF model can be equally useful for guiding the examination of PwMS or other neurologic disorders and impaired walking.

Given the high prevalence of imbalance and falls in PwMS, we recommend that balance and fall measures be used consistently in clinical and research settings to optimize clinical care, track disease progression, and assess response to disease-modifying and symptomatic intervention. Most of these measures are simple to use and provide high predictive value, as well as clinically and practically useful

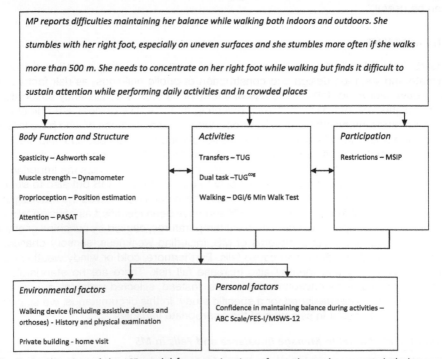

Fig. 3. Application of the ICF model for examination of a patient who reports imbalance or impaired walking.

information. These measures can identify problems at different levels of the ICF model and can then be used to direct interventions that will most effectively improve balance and reduce the risk of falls, as well as optimize independence, participation, and quality of life in PwMS.

REFERENCES

1. National Multiple Sclerosis Society. FAQs about MS. 2012. Available at: http://www. nationalmssociety.org/about-multiple-sclerosis/what-we-know-about-ms/faqs-about-ms/index.aspx#whogets. Accessed January 18, 2012.
2. Spain RI, St George RJ, Salarian A, et al. Body-worn motion sensors detect balance and gait deficits in people with multiple sclerosis who have normal walking speed. Gait Posture 2012;35:573–8.
3. Kalron A, Dvir Z, Achiron A. Effect of a cognitive task on postural control in patients with a clinically isolated syndrome suggestive of multiple sclerosis. Eur J Phys Rehabil Med 2011;47:579–86.
4. Nelson SR, Di Fabio RP, Anderson JH. Vestibular and sensory interaction deficits assessed by dynamic platform posturography in patients with multiple sclerosis. Ann Otol Rhinol Laryngol 1995;104:62–8.
5. Corradini ML, Fioretti S, Leo T, et al. Early recognition of postural disorders in multiple sclerosis through movement analysis: a modeling study. IEEE Trans Biomed Eng 1997;44:1029–38.
6. Karst GM, Venema DM, Roehrs TG, et al. Center of pressure measures during standing tasks in minimally impaired persons with multiple sclerosis. J Neurol Phys Ther 2005;29:170–80.
7. Martin CL, Phillips BA, Kilpatrick TJ, et al. Gait and balance impairment in early multiple sclerosis in the absence of clinical disability. Mult Scler 2006;12:620–8.
8. Jackson RT, Epstein CM, De l'Aune WR. Abnormalities in posturography and estimations of visual vertical and horizontal in multiple sclerosis. Am J Otol 1995;16:88–93.
9. Soyuer F, Mirza M, Erkorkmaz U. Balance performance in three forms of multiple sclerosis. Neurol Res 2006;28:555–62.
10. Cattaneo D, Jonsdottir J. Sensory impairments in quiet standing in subjects with multiple sclerosis. Mult Scler 2009;15:59–67.
11. Cattaneo D, Ferrarin M, Jonsdottir J, et al. The virtual time to contact in the evaluation of balance disorders and prediction of falls in people with multiple sclerosis. Disabil Rehabil 2012;34:470–7.
12. Jacobs JV, Kasser SL. Effects of dual tasking on the postural performance of people with and without multiple sclerosis: a pilot study. J Neurol 2012;259: 1166–76.
13. Cameron MH, Horak FB, Herndon RR, et al. Imbalance in multiple sclerosis: a result of slowed spinal somatosensory conduction. Somatosens Mot Res 2008;25:113–22.
14. Ramdharry GM, Marsden JF, Day BL, et al. De-stabilizing and training effects of foot orthoses in multiple sclerosis. Mult Scler 2006;12:219–26.
15. Rougier P, Thoumie P, Cantalloube S, et al. What compensatory motor strategies do patients with multiple sclerosis develop for balance control?. Rev Neurol (Paris) 2007;163:1054–64 [in French].
16. Chung LH, Remelius JG, Van Emmerik RE, et al. Leg power asymmetry and postural control in women with multiple sclerosis. Med Sci Sports Exerc 2008; 40:1717–24.

17. Frzovic D, Morris ME, Vowels L. Clinical tests of standing balance: performance of persons with multiple sclerosis. Arch Phys Med Rehabil 2000;81:215–21.
18. Remelius JG, Hamill J, Kent-Braun J, et al. Gait initiation in multiple sclerosis. Motor Control 2008;12:93–108.
19. Diener HC, Dichgans J, Hulser PJ, et al. The significance of delayed long-loop responses to ankle displacement for the diagnosis of multiple sclerosis. Electroencephalogr Clin Neurophysiol 1984;57:336–42.
20. Williams NP, Roland PS, Yellin W. Vestibular evaluation in patients with early multiple sclerosis. Am J Otol 1997;18:93–100.
21. Daley ML, Swank RL. Changes in postural control and vision induced by multiple sclerosis. Agressologie 1983;24:327–9.
22. Cattaneo D, De Nuzzo C, Fascia T, et al. Risks of falls in subjects with multiple sclerosis. Arch Phys Med Rehabil 2002;83:864–7.
23. Finlayson ML, Peterson EW, Cho CC. Risk factors for falling among people aged 45 to 90 years with multiple sclerosis. Arch Phys Med Rehabil 2006;87:1274–9.
24. Kasser SL, Jacobs JV, Foley JT, et al. A prospective evaluation of balance, gait, and strength to predict falling in women with multiple sclerosis. Arch Phys Med Rehabil 2011;92:1840–6.
25. Matsuda PN, Shumway-Cook A, Bamer AM, et al. Falls in multiple sclerosis. PM R 2011;3:624–32 [quiz: 32].
26. Nilsagard Y, Lundholm C, Denison E, et al. Predicting accidental falls in people with multiple sclerosis–a longitudinal study. Clin Rehabil 2009;23:259–69.
27. Sosnoff JJ, Socie MJ, Boes MK, et al. Mobility, balance and falls in persons with multiple sclerosis. PLoS One 2011;6:e28021.
28. Cameron MH, Poel AJ, Haselkorn JK, et al. Falls requiring medical attention among veterans with multiple sclerosis: a cohort study. J Rehabil Res Dev 2011;48:13–20.
29. Matsuda PN, Shumway-Cook A, Ciol MA, et al. Understanding falls in multiple sclerosis: association of mobility status, concerns about falling, and accumulated impairments. Phys Ther 2012;92:407–15.
30. Peterson EW, Cho CC, Finlayson ML. Fear of falling and associated activity curtailment among middle aged and older adults with multiple sclerosis. Mult Scler 2007;13:1168–75.
31. Peterson EW, Cho CC, von Koch L, et al. Injurious falls among middle aged and older adults with multiple sclerosis. Arch Phys Med Rehabil 2008;89:1031–7.
32. Moen SM, Celius EG, Nordsletten L, et al. Fractures and falls in patients with newly diagnosed clinically isolated syndrome and multiple sclerosis. Acta Neurol Scand Suppl 2011;(191):79–82.
33. Bazelier MT, de Vries F, Bentzen J, et al. Incidence of fractures in patients with multiple sclerosis: the Danish National Health Registers. Mult Scler 2012;18: 622–77.
34. Motl RW, Snook EM, Agiovlasitis S, et al. Calibration of accelerometer output for ambulatory adults with multiple sclerosis. Arch Phys Med Rehabil 2009;90:1778–84.
35. Daley ML, Swank RL. Quantitative posturography: use in multiple sclerosis. IEEE Trans Biomed Eng 1981;28:668–71.
36. Pratt CA, Horak FB, Herndon RM. Differential effects of somatosensory and motor system deficits on postural dyscontrol in multiple sclerosis patients. In: Woollacoot M, Horak FB, editors. Posture and gait: control mechanisms. Portland (OR): University of Oregon Books; 1992. p. 118–21.
37. Sosnoff JJ, Shin S, Motl RW. Multiple sclerosis and postural control: the role of spasticity. Arch Phys Med Rehabil 2010;91:93–9.

38. Sosnoff JJ, Gappmaier E, Frame A, et al. Influence of spasticity on mobility and balance in persons with multiple sclerosis. J Neurol Phys Ther 2011;35:129–32.
39. Nilsagard Y, Denison E, Gunnarsson LG, et al. Factors perceived as being related to accidental falls by persons with multiple sclerosis. Disabil Rehabil 2009;31:1301–10.
40. World Health Organization. International classification of functioning, disability and health (ICF). Geneva (Switzerland): World Health Organization; 2001.
41. Kurtzke JF. Rating neurologic impairment in multiple sclerosis: an expanded disability status scale (EDSS). Neurology 1983;33:1444–52.
42. Cutter GR, Baier ML, Rudick RA, et al. Development of a multiple sclerosis functional composite as a clinical trial outcome measure. Brain 1999;122:871–82.
43. Goodkin DE, Cookfair D, Wende K, et al. Inter- and intrarater scoring agreement using grades 1.0 to 3.5 of the Kurtzke Expanded Disability Status Scale (EDSS). Multiple Sclerosis Collaborative Research Group. Neurology 1992;42:859–63.
44. Sharrack B, Hughes RA, Soudain S, et al. The psychometric properties of clinical rating scales used in multiple sclerosis. Brain 1999;122(Pt 1):141–59.
45. Prosperini L, Leonardi L, De Carli P, et al. Visuo-proprioceptive training reduces risk of falls in patients with multiple sclerosis. Mult Scler 2010;16:491–9.
46. Bohannon RW, Smith MB. Interrater reliability of a modified Ashworth scale of muscle spasticity. Phys Ther 1987;67:206–7.
47. Benedetti MG, Piperno R, Simoncini L, et al. Gait abnormalities in minimally impaired multiple sclerosis patients. Mult Scler 1999;5:363–8.
48. Kelleher KJ, Spence W, Solomonidis S, et al. The characterisation of gait patterns of people with multiple sclerosis. Disabil Rehabil 2010;32:1242–50.
49. Givon U, Zeilig G, Achiron A. Gait analysis in multiple sclerosis: characterization of temporal-spatial parameters using GAITRite functional ambulation system. Gait Posture 2009;29:138–42.
50. van Uden CJ, Besser MP. Test-retest reliability of temporal and spatial gait characteristics measured with an instrumented walkway system (GAITRite). BMC Musculoskelet Disord 2004;5:13.
51. Elbers RG, Rietberg MB, van Wegen EE, et al. Self-report fatigue questionnaires in multiple sclerosis, Parkinson's disease and stroke: a systematic review of measurement properties. Qual Life Res 2012;21:925–44.
52. Penner IK, Raselli C, Stocklin M, et al. The Fatigue Scale for Motor and Cognitive Functions (FSMC): validation of a new instrument to assess multiple sclerosis-related fatigue. Mult Scler 2009;15:1509–17.
53. Doward LC, Meads DM, Fisk J, et al. International development of the Unidimensional Fatigue Impact Scale (U-FIS). Value Health 2010;13:463–8.
54. Meads DM, Doward LC, McKenna SP, et al. The development and validation of the Unidimensional Fatigue Impact Scale (U-FIS). Mult Scler 2009;15:1228–38.
55. Krupp LB, LaRocca NG, Muir-Nash J, et al. The fatigue severity scale. Application to patients with multiple sclerosis and systemic lupus erythematosus. Arch Neurol 1989;46:1121–3.
56. Flachenecker P, Kumpfel T, Kallmann B, et al. Fatigue in multiple sclerosis: a comparison of different rating scales and correlation to clinical parameters. Mult Scler 2002;8:523–6.
57. Zifko UA, Rupp M, Schwarz S, et al. Modafinil in treatment of fatigue in multiple sclerosis. Results of an open-label study. J Neurol 2002;249:983–7.
58. Rammohan KW, Rosenberg JH, Lynn DJ, et al. Efficacy and safety of modafinil (Provigil) for the treatment of fatigue in multiple sclerosis: a two centre phase 2 study. J Neurol Neurosurg Psychiatry 2002;72:179–83.

59. Negahban H, Mofateh R, Arastoo AA, et al. The effects of cognitive loading on balance control in patients with multiple sclerosis. Gait Posture 2011;34:479–84.
60. Hamilton F, Rochester L, Paul L, et al. Walking and talking: an investigation of cognitive-motor dual tasking in multiple sclerosis. Mult Scler 2009;15:1215–27.
61. Boes MK, Sosnoff JJ, Socie MJ, et al. Postural control in multiple sclerosis: effects of disability status and dual task. J Neurol Sci 2012;315:44–8.
62. Sosnoff JJ, Boes MK, Sandroff BM, et al. Walking and thinking in persons with multiple sclerosis who vary in disability. Arch Phys Med Rehabil 2011;92:2028–33.
63. Benedict RH, Cookfair D, Gavett R, et al. Validity of the minimal assessment of cognitive function in multiple sclerosis (MACFIMS). J Int Neuropsychol Soc 2006;12:549–58.
64. Langdon D, Amato M, Boringa J, et al. Recommendations for a Brief International Cognitive Assessment for Multiple Sclerosis (BICAMS). Mult Scler 2012; 18:891–8.
65. Lord SR, Menz HB, Tiedemann A. A physiological profile approach to falls risk assessment and prevention. Phys Ther 2003;83:237–52.
66. Podsiadlo D, Richardson S. The timed "Up & Go": a test of basic functional mobility for frail elderly persons. J Am Geriatr Soc 1991;39:142–8.
67. Nilsagård Y, Lundholm C, Gunnarsson LG, et al. Clinical relevance using timed walk tests and 'timed up and go' testing in persons with multiple sclerosis. Physiother Res Int 2007;12:105–14.
68. Learmonth YC, Paul L, McFadyen AK, et al. Reliability and clinical significance of mobility and balance assessments in multiple sclerosis. Int J Rehabil Res 2012;35:69–74.
69. Cattaneo D, Regola A, Meotti M. Validity of six balance disorders scales in persons with multiple sclerosis. Disabil Rehabil 2006;28:789–95.
70. Isles RC, Choy NL, Steer M, et al. Normal values of balance tests in women aged 20-80. J Am Geriatr Soc 2004;52:1367–72.
71. Shumway-Cook A, Brauer S, Woollacott M. Predicting the probability for falls in community-dwelling older adults using the Timed Up & Go Test. Phys Ther 2000; 80:896–903.
72. Steffen TM, Hacker TA, Mollinger L. Age- and gender-related test performance in community-dwelling elderly people: Six-Minute Walk Test, Berg Balance Scale, Timed Up & Go Test, and gait speeds. Phys Ther 2002;82:128–37.
73. Berg K, Wood-Dauphinee S, Williams JI, et al. Measuring balance in the elderly: preliminary development of an instrument. Physiother Can 1989;41:304–11.
74. Cattaneo D, Jonsdottir J, Repetti S. Reliability of four scales on balance disorders in persons with multiple sclerosis. Disabil Rehabil 2007;29:1920–5.
75. McConvey J, Bennett SE. Reliability of the Dynamic Gait Index in individuals with multiple sclerosis. Arch Phys Med Rehabil 2005;86:130–3.
76. Duncan PW, Weiner DK, Chandler J, et al. Functional reach: a new clinical measure of balance. J Gerontol 1990;45:M192–7.
77. Dite W, Temple VA. A clinical test of stepping and change of direction to identify multiple falling older adults. Arch Phys Med Rehabil 2002;83:1566–71.
78. Horak FB, Wrisley DM, Frank J. The Balance Evaluation Systems Test (BESTest) to differentiate balance deficits. Phys Ther 2009;89:484–98.
79. Franchignoni F, Horak F, Godi M, et al. Using psychometric techniques to improve the Balance Evaluation Systems Test: the mini-BESTest. J Rehabil Med 2010;42:323–31.
80. Schwid SR, Goodman AD, McDermott MP, et al. Quantitative functional measures in MS: what is a reliable change? Neurology 2002;58:1294–6.

81. Goldman MD, Marrie RA, Cohen JA. Evaluation of the six-minute walk in multiple sclerosis subjects and healthy controls. Mult Scler 2008;14:383–90.

82. Goldman MD, Motl RW, Rudick RA. Possible clinical outcome measures for clinical trials in patients with multiple sclerosis. Ther Adv Neurol Disord 2010;3: 229–39.

83. Holper L, Coenen M, Weise A, et al. Characterization of functioning in multiple sclerosis using the ICF. J Neurol 2010;257:103–13.

84. Gijbels D, Dalgas U, Romberg A, et al. Which walking capacity tests to use in multiple sclerosis? A multicentre study providing the basis for a core set. Mult Scler 2012;18:364–71.

85. Yasui NY, Berven NL. Community integration: conceptualisation and measurement. Disabil Rehabil 2009;31:761–71.

86. Cardol M, de Haan RJ, van den Bos GA, et al. The development of a handicap assessment questionnaire: the Impact on Participation and Autonomy (IPA). Clin Rehabil 1999;13:411–9.

87. Willer B, Ottenbacher KJ, Coad ML. The community integration questionnaire. A comparative examination. Am J Phys Med Rehabil 1994;73:103–11.

88. Gontkovsky ST, Russum P, Stokic DS. Comparison of the CIQ and CHART Short Form in assessing community integration in individuals with chronic spinal cord injury: a pilot study. NeuroRehabilitation 2009;24:185–92.

89. Ehde DM, Osborne TL, Hanley MA, et al. The scope and nature of pain in persons with multiple sclerosis. Mult Scler 2006;12:629–38.

90. Hirsh AT, Braden AL, Craggs JG, et al. Psychometric properties of the community integration questionnaire in a heterogeneous sample of adults with physical disability. Arch Phys Med Rehabil 2011;92:1602–10.

91. Walker N, Mellick D, Brooks CA, et al. Measuring participation across impairment groups using the Craig Handicap Assessment Reporting Technique. Am J Phys Med Rehabil 2003;82:936–41.

92. Wynia K, Middel B, van Dijk JP, et al. The Multiple Sclerosis impact Profile (MSIP). Development and testing psychometric properties of an ICF-based health measure. Disabil Rehabil 2008;30:261–74.

93. Wynia K, Middel B, de Ruiter H, et al. Stability and relative validity of the Multiple Sclerosis Impact Profile (MSIP). Disabil Rehabil 2008;30:1027–38.

94. Powell LE, Myers AM. The Activities-specific Balance Confidence (ABC) Scale. J Gerontol A Biol Sci Med Sci 1995;50A:M28–34.

95. Nilsagard Y, Carling A, Forsberg A. Activities-specific balance confidence in people with multiple sclerosis. Mult Scler Int 2012;2012:613925.

96. Jacobson GP, Newman CW. The development of the Dizziness Handicap Inventory. Arch Otolaryngol Head Neck Surg 1990;116:424–7.

97. Tinetti ME, Richman D, Powell L. Falls efficacy as a measure of fear of falling. J Gerontol 1990;45:P239–43.

98. Yardley L, Beyer N, Hauer K, et al. Development and initial validation of the Falls Efficacy Scale-International (FES-I). Age Ageing 2005;34:614–9.

99. Hauer K, Yardley L, Beyer N, et al. Validation of the Falls Efficacy Scale and Falls Efficacy Scale International in geriatric patients with and without cognitive impairment: results of self-report and interview-based questionnaires. Gerontology 2010;56:190–9.

100. Hobart JC, Riazi A, Lamping DL, et al. Measuring the impact of MS on walking ability: the 12-Item MS Walking Scale (MSWS-12). Neurology 2003;60:31–6.

101. McGuigan C, Hutchinson M. Confirming the validity and responsiveness of the Multiple Sclerosis Walking Scale-12 (MSWS-12). Neurology 2004;62:2103–5.

102. Motl RW, Snook EM. Confirmation and extension of the validity of the Multiple Sclerosis Walking Scale-12 (MSWS-12). J Neurol Sci 2008;268:69–73.
103. Nilsagård Y, Gunnarsson L, Denison E. Self-perceived limitations of gait in persons with multiple sclerosis. Adv Physiother 2007;9:136–43.
104. McGuigan C, Hutchinson M. The multiple sclerosis impact scale (MSIS-29) is a reliable and sensitive measure. J Neurol Neurosurg Psychiatry 2004;75:266–9.
105. Nilsagård Y, Forsberg A. Psychometric properties of the Activities-Specific Balance Confidence Scale in persons 0-14 days and 3 months post stroke. Disabil Rehabil 2012;34:1186–91.
106. Gold SM, Schulz H, Monch A, et al. Cognitive impairment in multiple sclerosis does not affect reliability and validity of self-report health measures. Mult Scler 2003;9:404–10.

Ambulation and Spinal Cord Injury

Elizabeth C. Hardin, PhD[a,b,*], Rudi Kobetic, MSBE[a],
Ronald J. Triolo, PhD[a,b,c]

KEYWORDS

- Spinal cord injury • Ambulation • Walking • Rehabilitation • Treadmill • Stimulation

KEY POINTS

- Muscle atrophy and bone loss accompany spinal cord injuries (SCI), but walking promotes musculoskeletal health, reduces inflammation, and can enhance mental health.
- Walking is possible for many with an SCI; but clarify whether walking is for exercise, activities of daily living, community ambulation, or to fulfill a psychological need to walk.
- Devices that enable walking include braces, body-weight-supported treadmills, functional electrical stimulation (FES), robotic-assisted devices, and hybrid devices. Robotic-assisted treadmills improve function similar to other approaches.
- The primary outcome measures for walking recovery and capacity are the Walking Index for SCI II, 10-minute walk test, 6-minute walk test, and Spinal Cord Independence Measure. For measuring community ambulation, the Spinal Cord Functional Ambulation Profile is recommended.
- Continued walking may be limited by many factors, including inaccessibility, shoulder pain, falling injuries, medications, and unrealistic expectations. Use strategies to address these if accompanied by negative changes in quality of life.

WHY IS WALKING IMPORTANT AFTER SPINAL CORD INJURY?

Spinal cord injuries (SCI) cause the degradation or loss of walking ability, along with mechanical unloading of the lower extremities resulting in profound muscle atrophy and bone loss. Walking provides exercise that promotes musculoskeletal health, reduces systemic inflammation, enhances mental health, enables community involvement, and can make the activities of daily living more efficient. Unfortunately, accompanying these benefits are potential negative consequences of walking, including the risk of falling, dissatisfaction related to unrealistic expectations, and even negative

[a] Motion Study Laboratory, Louis Stokes Cleveland VA Medical Center, 10701 East Boulevard, Cleveland, OH 44106, USA; [b] Department of Biomedical Engineering, Case Western Reserve University, 319 Wickenden Building, 10900 Euclid Avenue, Cleveland, OH 44106-7207, USA; [c] Department of Orthopaedics, Case School of Medicine/University Hospitals, 11100 Euclid Avenue, Cleveland, OH 44106-5043, USA
* Corresponding author. Motion Study Laboratory, Cleveland VA Medical Center, 151A, 10701 East Boulevard, Cleveland, OH 44106.
E-mail address: ehardin@fescenter.org

Phys Med Rehabil Clin N Am 24 (2013) 355–370
http://dx.doi.org/10.1016/j.pmr.2012.11.002
1047-9651/13/$ – see front matter Published by Elsevier Inc.

pmr.theclinics.com

changes in quality of life. Regaining walking function is one critical goal during the rehabilitation period, but the goals and process for regaining the ability to walk should be clearly addressed with patients, including whether walking is regained for daily function or for exercise only.

Systemic Inflammation

High systemic inflammation is related to a high body mass index, a history of pressure ulcers, and urinary tract infections, which are all common consequences of SCI, and can be moderated with regular walking exercise. Cardiovascular health can also be influenced by systemic inflammation and moderated with walking exercise. Inflammation has been independently related to the mode of locomotion in individuals with chronic SCI.[1] In this study, inflammation was lowest in those who walked with an assistive device, walked independently, or used a manual wheelchair.

Muscle Loading

Load bearing by the lower extremities increases muscle activity in those with SCI as reflected in the amplitude of electromyography (EMG), possibly because of sensory input.[2] Based on these observations, minimizing upper limb loading with handrails or parallel bars, while increasing vertical load bearing through the legs, should be encouraged during walking. This practice has been translated into a guiding principle for improving muscle activation in those muscles that are weak.

Cartilage Atrophy

In a study about cartilage health in those with SCI who were ambulators, capable of walking and not confined to their wheelchair, and those who were nonambulators, it was found that nonambulators with SCI experienced increased cartilage atrophy and degradation.[3] Articular cartilage degradation has been associated with elevated collagen type-II levels in individuals with SCI who are nonambulators or physiologic ambulators. The following factors can cause significant differences in collagen type-II levels: injury level Asia Impairment Scale (AIS) A (**Table 1**), a zero functional

Table 1
The 5 categories of the AIS represent different levels of presence or absence of sensory and motor function

AIS Categories	Sensory and Motor Function
A: Complete	No sensory or motor function is preserved in the sacral segments S4–S5.
B: Sensory Incomplete	Sensory but not motor function is preserved below the neurologic level and includes the sacral segments S4–S5 (light touch, pin prick at S4–S5 or deep anal pressure and no motor function is preserved more than 3 levels below the motor level on either side of the body).
C: Motor Incomplete	Motor function is preserved below the neurologic level, and more than half of the key muscle functions below the single neurologic level of injury have a muscle grade less than 3 (grades 0–2).
D: Motor Incomplete	Motor function is preserved below the neurologic level, and at least half (half or more) of the key muscle functions below the neurologic level of injury have a muscle grade greater than 3.
E: Normal	If sensation and motor function are graded as normal in all segments and patients had prior deficits, then the AIS grade is E. Someone without an initial SCI does not receive an AIS grade.

ambulation score, and little daily ambulation. Thus, therapy should be initiated as soon as possible after SCI to minimize cartilage atrophy.

Bone Density

Walking retains bone mineral content and should be started as early as possible in the postinjury phase to reduce mineral loss.[4] Nearly one-half of the mineral content below the lesion level is lost within the first year after injury, so walking is vital to bone health. Another recent study suggests that there is an association between circulating sclerostin and bone density in chronic SCI.[5] Sclerostin is a protein that is produced by the osteocyte; it has anti-anabolic effects on bone formation. Levels of sclerostin, a biomarker of osteoporosis severity, were reduced in patients with SCI who used a wheelchair compared with individuals with SCI who walked regularly. Circulating sclerostin was deemed a biomarker of osteoporosis severity in chronic paraplegia rather than a mediator of ongoing bone loss. This finding was in contrast to animal models of mechanical unloading whereby high sclerostin levels suppress bone formation acutely. Bone loss can also be asymmetric in the lower limbs because of walking asymmetries in patients with incomplete SCI (iSCI).[6]

Quality of Life

A change in mobility within the first year after injury can significantly impact perceived quality of life.[7] Individuals with SCI who transitioned from walking at discharge to wheelchair use have low quality-of-life indicators, including high pain and depression scores. The data suggest that marginal ambulators be encouraged to work toward functional independence from a wheelchair rather than depend on primary ambulation during acute rehabilitation. Self-help mental health programs should also be included for inpatient ambulators and those who are discharged as ambulators.[8] Some patients may also have unrealistic expectations about walking that may cause the activity to be abandoned, for example, that it will lead to complete recovery of walking function or recovery from SCI altogether.[9]

Clinical Decision Making

Understanding individual ambulation deficits is critical for clinical decision making[10] because many patients with iSCI require gait reeducation, especially for those at the AIS D level (see **Table 1**). The ambulation prognosis generally depends on muscle power loss, degree of spasticity, type of lower limb joint deformity developed, and availability of treatment. As an adjunct to physical examination and observation, gait analysis can inform treatment with measures of 3-dimensional dynamic joint range motion (kinematics) and estimation of joint forces (kinetics) at the hip, knee, and ankle. These measurements can be combined with walking EMG and energy cost measures to fully understand the gait disturbance.

MEASURING AND PREDICTING WALKING FUNCTION
Assessments to Measure Walking Function and Recovery

For many years, the initial level of injury and the severity of motor and sensory impairment were considered to reliably predict neurologic recovery of function after SCI; however, it is now known that using impairment scales to predict walking function is unrealistic. The AIS conversion outcome measure is poorly related to the ability to walk in patients with traumatic SCI (van Middendorp and colleagues,[11] 2009). Instead, composite measures are recommended to predict the recovery of walking capacity and function. Outcome measures have evolved to measure the effectiveness of newer activity-based therapies in clinical trials. For example, 6 different outcome measures were related to walking function improvement in a randomized clinical trial for walking plasticity after SCI[12]: (1) motor strength; (2) balance; (3) Walking Index for SCI (WISCI); (4) walking speed; (5) 6-minute walk (walking capacity); and (6) locomotor functional independence measure (FIM), a disability measure. An effort is currently underway to develop a more contemporary functional outcome measure for use in SCI research, which will eventually lead to the SCI computer adaptive test. Functional activities that are important to patients with SCI have been selected using focus group discussions comprised of patients with SCI and clinical staff conducted at 6 US National Spinal Cord Injury Model Systems Programs.[13] The item pool included 326 functional activity items fitting into categories from the International Classification of Functioning, Disability, and Health framework. This item pool is being field tested to develop a calibrated item bank.

Measuring the progress of walking through recovery or reeducation therapy requires using measures that standardize injury severity and walking capacity. Standardized severity measures are detailed in the 2011 International Standards for Neurologic Classification of SCI, the clinical gold standard.[14] Measurements of walking capacity have evolved into valid, reliable, and responsive instruments, including the WISCI II; the Spinal Cord Independence Measure (SCIM); the Spinal Cord Functional Ambulation Profile (SCI-FAP); and timed tests, such as the 10-minute walk test (10MWT) and the 6-minute walk test (6MWT). These measurements are necessary for understanding recovery mechanisms and for separating neurologic improvement from adaptation through rehabilitation.[15,16]

Baseline examination accuracy is especially critical in the acute phase of injury for determining spontaneous walking recovery. Categorical scales, such as the WISCI, generally have floor and ceiling effects, whereas timed measures have excellent reliability, construct validity, and responsiveness to change in measuring SCI walking function.[17] The psychometric properties of these measures are variable, although those developed specifically for the SCI population have excellent reliability and validity.[18] Eight disability outcome measures have been evaluated for acute traumatic SCI. The SCIM had validity and responsiveness and was the best *comprehensive* measure of functional recovery during rehabilitation, even after discharge.[19] These findings were endorsed by The Spinal Cord Injury Solutions Network.[18] Although initially after the injury, walking capacity and the SCIM mobility items were moderately correlated, the correlations improved at 6 and 12 months.[19] When the patients were divided by injury level, the mobility items were only initially responsive for those at levels AIS A and B. For those at level AIS C and D, the SCIM had responsiveness during the first 6 months; furthermore, the correlation with walking capacity increased over time after injury in those with AIS C but decreased in those with AIS D. In addition, walking capacity was more highly correlated with indoor mobility compared with outdoor mobility. Although the WISCI has validity and reliability for those with acute SCI, more psychometric studies are needed for those with chronic SCI.[20–22] In addition, some WISCI II categories are redundant and the test has ceiling effects that limit its usefulness.[23]

Timed walking tests, specifically the Timed Up and Go (TUG), the 10MWT, and the 6MWT, are valid and reliable measures for assessing walking function.[17,24] The reliability of the TUG and 10MWT is negatively influenced by poor walking function, as assessed in a group of 75 patients.[23] Furthermore, although the relationship between the TUG and the 10MWT was strong, it changed over time. In addition, this study revealed that the WISCI II had internal redundancy. The best measure to assess walking capacity was determined to be the 10MWT; but it was advised that a walking endurance measure be included, such as the 6MWT.[22] In another study, the 10MWT and the WISCI II were used effectively to evaluate the efficacy of walking rehabilitation programs.[25]

The primary outcome measures for walking recovery and capacity are, thus, the WISCI II, 10MWT, 6MWT, and SCIM.[18,19,22] For measuring community ambulation function, the SCI-FAP should be used because it incorporates the timed performance of 7 tasks, including walking and negotiating obstacles, doors, and stairs.[16]

Walking Function Recovery

In those with motor iSCI, a combination of parameters gives a reliable prediction of walking stratification.[26] Eleven measures from the subacute injury period were related to ambulatory outcome measures 6 months after injury, including clinical examination, tibial somatosensory evoked potentials (tSSEP), and demographic factors. The Lower Extremity Motor Score (LEMS), in combination with other measures, can predict walking at a later stage. However, the percentage of correct predictions in patients with paraparesis was lower for those who had a poor walking outcome. The authors' clinical algorithm also identified a subgroup of patients with tetraparesis and poor ambulatory recovery. The following algorithms were determined:

Paraparesis algorithms
    WISCI II prediction $Z = -13.39 + 0.1(LEMS) + 0.12$ (pin prick*)
    *Using AIS as the second factor provided similar predictions.
    6-minute walk prediction $Z = -0.28 + 0.28(LEMS) - 0.09$ (age**)
    **Adding age as the second factor did not increase the percentage of correct
        predictions but did improve the goodness of fit.

Tetraparesis algorithms
    WISCI II prediction $Z = -10.96 + 0.28$ (LEMS) $+ 1.51$ (minimum tSSEP)
    6-minute walk prediction $Z = -354.02 + 10.24$ (LEMS) $+ 61.96$ (AIS)

Muscle Strength

After an iSCI, those with relatively preserved leg muscle strength have a greater chance for improvements in walking speed after locomotor training (Yang and colleagues,[27] 2011). Lower extremity muscle strength, measured with the manual muscle test can identify key muscle groups related to walking speed improvements. These groups were the knee extensors, knee flexors, ankle plantar flexors, and hip abductors. Although these results are exploratory, they suggested that preserved muscle strength in the legs after iSCI would predict speed improvements after locomotor training. Quadriceps strength alone can be a predictor of walking function. Crozier and colleagues[28] found that patients with motor incomplete injuries who recovered quadriceps strength of greater than 3/5 by 2 months after injury, as tested by the manual muscle test, had an excellent prognosis for ambulation at 6 months. The 3/5 value signified that they could flex and extend the knee against gravity without manual resistance where 5/5 would be normal function. They defined functional ambulators as those patients who were able to walk in the household and/or the community; nonambulators were those who did not ambulate or did so only for exercise.

Cause

Functional outcome may depend on SCI cause, thus comparisons were made between individuals with inflammatory myelopathies and traumatic spinal cord lesions.[29] This study showed that the functional outcome was determined by lesion level, severity, and age rather than by cause. On the other hand, in a study of elderly patients with nontraumatic SCI, differences based on cause were found in rehabilitation length of stay and functional outcomes.[30] Patients with degenerative spinal disease and benign tumors had a higher frequency of independent walking than patients with malignant tumors or spinal abscess, and they had the shortest rehabilitation period. Furthermore, patients with vascular ischemia were less likely to be independent in their walking than those with degenerative spinal disease and benign tumor, and they had the longest rehabilitation period. Finally, a study of 70 adults with nontraumatic SCI undergoing initial inpatient rehabilitation found that disability was significantly reduced during rehabilitation, with 76% discharged home.[31] Of those discharged home, 15% walked unaided, 43% walked at least 10 m with a walking aid, while 42% were wheelchair dependent.

Age and Gender

In patients with nontraumatic SCI, age and gender do not significantly influence most aspects of walking rehabilitation.[32] The only complication that was related to age was pressure ulcers. Age should not discriminate those who will benefit from walking rehabilitation, and individuals with chronic iSCI can also benefit from rehabilitation (Gorgey and colleagues,[33] 2010). Even a twice-weekly dose of body-weight-supported treadmill training (BWSTT) can promote motor recovery for walking when accompanied with resistance training. For example, 10 weeks of BWSTT and resistance training for the knee extensor muscles can enhance walking function as found in one case study. Initially, the patient was a short-distance ambulator (<50 ft) who primarily relied on a power wheelchair and, after training, recovered the independent use of bilateral crutches to walk 200 ft and increased their overground walking speed. The FIM locomotion score increased from 3 to 6, the Berg balance score increased from 11 to 41, and the WISCI score increased from 1 to 10. Three months after discharge, independent functional walking was maintained.

Independence and Walking

The ability to walk might be associated with greater independence and well-being after an SCI. In investigating the association of the locomotion mode with health and well-being, Krause and colleagues[34] found associations between locomotion independence and every health and well-being outcome, whereas nonindependent, nonambulators had poor health and well-being outcomes. Those who ambulated did not, however, uniformly report better outcomes than wheelchair users. For example, those who depended on others for walking assistance had less favorable outcomes.

Weighing the Risks and Benefits of Walking

Along with the benefits from walking are accompanying risks. The problems encountered by those who walk in the SCI population range from shoulder pain to an increased risk of falling. Shoulder pain is typically thought to be related to manual wheelchair use; but in those with chronic SCI, the prevalence of shoulder pain was 33.3% in participants walking without assistance; 47.6% in participants using crutches, canes, or walkers; 46.7% in motorized wheelchair users; and 35.4% in manual wheelchair users.[35] It is, therefore, critical to assess the mechanical and nonmechanical factors that can lead to shoulder pain. Walking can also increase the risk of falls and must be addressed with patients. Brotherton and colleagues[36] identified factors that were independently associated with having had a fall in the past year. The odds of falling were lower with those who had better current perceived health, those who had better perceived health compared with a year ago, individuals who exercised more frequently, and those who used a walker. In addition, the fear of falling, or the self-perception of confidence as measured by the Modified Falls Efficacy Scale, might not be an accurate representation of postural stability in those with low-level paraplegia who walk with bilateral knee-ankle-foot orthoses. The Modified Falls Efficacy Scale was negatively correlated with postural control, suggesting that this scale does not reflect postural control as measured during walking in this population.[37] Clinicians should, thus, consider fear of falling as an influential factor in postural control during rehabilitation.

IMPROVING WALKING

There are numerous modalities to improve walking. Initially, walking deficits must be determined, either observationally or, more accurately, with gait analysis, to design a targeted rehabilitation program. Walking may be improved with task-oriented therapies, such as overground walking or BWSTT, which can include sensory input or reflex training. Orthoses that use FES, robotics, and/or bracing are at the forefront of technologies that enable those with SCI to walk. FES gives patients the opportunity to perform exercises for specific muscle groups, in addition to facilitating walking. Well-controlled studies exist that compare various walking modalities; but clinical practicability, effectiveness, and cost-efficiency were not systematically assessed.

Gait Analysis Defines Walking Deficits

A gait analysis assessment results in a customized plan for walking rehabilitation. Gait analysis can be used effectively, especially in patients at the AIS D level.[10,12,38] The measures range from spatiotemporal parameters of gait (eg, speed, cadence, and stride length) to measurements from 3-dimensional motion analysis systems and multichannel EMG. An observational gait analysis by a clinician can determine walking impairments following iSCI; the most common of these are inadequate hip extension during stance, persistent plantar flexion, decreased hip/knee flexion during swing, and inadequate foot placement at initial contact of the stance phase. Walking prognosis will, however, depend on muscle power loss, spasticity, and lower limb joint deformity. To accurately determine deficits, an instrumented gait analysis, including measurements of 3-dimensional kinematics and kinetics (joint forces, moments, and powers providing information on muscle actions), is needed and can be combined with EMG and energy cost to determine how contractures and muscular deficits influence the limb during walking. The deficits differ widely between those with iSCI; but for those with thoracic lesions, the angular velocity of the knee is generally slower, whereas for those with lumbar lesions, the angular velocity of the ankle is generally slower.[39] Also, at initial contact, there is greater hip abduction than in able-bodied individuals; but at foot-off, there is less hip abduction, which persists during swing, hampering limb clearance.[40]

Gait analysis has dramatically changed spasticity management in children with cerebral palsy by guiding surgical and other treatments. Gait analysis can also direct a task-oriented approach for training walking or a sensorimotor intervention. Moreover, those responding to a sensorimotor intervention can be rapidly identified with gait analysis.[38] Dynamic energy cost estimations could also be used as an outcome to study improvements after treatment, whether the treatment is physical therapy, surgery, pharmacology, an orthosis, or a combination of these treatments. Unfortunately, the cost/benefit ratio of using gait analysis for improving walking function in those with iSCI is unknown.

Recovery of Walking Through Activity-Based Therapies

Physical rehabilitation strategies such as activity-based therapies can improve recovery from iSCI beyond the initial prognosis.[2] Training strategies using BWSTT and manual assistance are being used more frequently; the first prospective, multi-center, randomized clinical trial using a task-oriented walking intervention was administrated by Dobkin and colleagues.[41] Developing evidence-based practices was the purpose behind this trial for patients with acute SCI.[41,42] The methodology was developed for those within 8 weeks of injury, and 146 patients received 12 weeks of therapy. Primary outcome measures were the level of walking independence and the maximal speed for walking 50 ft at 12 weeks and 6 and 12 months. After 12 weeks of BWSTT, most AIS C and D participants achieved functional walking, although few AIS A patients reached this category.[42] Recently, BWSTT outcomes were revealed to be similar to those of overground training, thus time- and personnel-intensive BWSTT training may not be warranted.[43] In fact, a review of 4 randomized clinical trials showed that one walking training strategy does not improve walking more than another strategy when comparing conventional gait training with BWSTT.[44] In AIS C patients whereby flexor activity predominates, load-bearing activity-based therapies can promote extensor activity during the stance phase.[2]

Walking speed can be improved in those with chronic iSCI with activity-based therapies.[45] Walking ability and psychological well-being improved in 35 adults with chronic iSCI for more than 1 year (AIS C and AIS D), both with BWSTT and walking in a fixed track device with body-weight support. Improved walking speed was associated with increased balance and muscle strength. The outcomes were similar to those of individuals with iSCI receiving comprehensive physical therapy for improving walking speed and strength.

Reflex Training and Walking

Appropriate reflex conditioning improves walking in rats after SCI[46]; in humans, there is evidence to support this phenomenon, although the changes seem to occur within the first 3 months after injury.[47,48] This finding could be caused by better gating of peripheral afferent feedback. Some patients with iSCI had preserved mechanisms for cyclic soleus H-reflex modulation during walking with body weight support (BWS) loads of 35% to 60%, whereas in others there was an absent H-reflex depression during the swing phase.[47] The best evidence of reflex conditioning comes from a study of 2 groups of patients with iSCI: those who were either less than 3 months after injury or 3 to 12 months after injury.[48] Transcranial magnetic stimulation was used to assess soleus H-reflex modulation. Patients that were less than 3 months after injury exhibited an increase in H reflex facilitation at 20 milliseconds, an increased gait velocity, and a positive correlation with the WISCI II compared with those who were more than 3 months after injury. Reflex modulation was postulated to change in the first 3 months after injury. Other pathways may also be altered by these conditioning protocols, such as reciprocal inhibition.

FES with BWSTT

In addition to the factors described earlier, the potential for recovering walking depends on the intervention type, duration, and specificity, and whether interventions are combined. With the immediate application of FES or BWSTT, there is a gradient of effects, from small changes with the immediate application to larger changes when combined with pharmacologic approaches.[49] Walking-specific training should be optimized to maximally exploit spontaneous and induced neural plasticity.[25] In comparing BWSTT with or without FES or robotic-assisted step training (RAST), using walking speed and capacity as outcomes, either locomotor training strategy was noted to improve walking.[44] After the period of spontaneous recovery, FES combined with BWSTT can improve walking; but few controlled studies exist.[50] FES with BWSTT may have physiologic and psychological benefits that would justify their use in acute and chronic SCI populations.[51] Unfortunately, access to BWSTT and walking training with FES is restricted under managed care, so patients with chronic SCI usually do not have access to these options. Recently, however, one study enrolled 64 patients with chronic iSCI and had them train for 5 days per week for 12 weeks using (1) treadmill training with manual assistance; (2) treadmill training with FES; (3) treadmill training with robotic assistance, but without active participation; or (4) overground training with FES.[52] Patients improved their speed with overground training or treadmill-based training, but distance improved to a greater extent with overground training and FES. There was no evidence for an optimal training dosage and speed. Retesting 10 patients 6 months after training showed that speed had slowed compared with after training but was faster than before training. Lastly, the training of supraspinal control, such as attention demands and visual input, should be considered. These areas are essential in human locomotion; for those with iSCI, they may be critical because an increased falling risk was shown to be influenced by poor supraspinal control.[25] The iSCI population depends greatly on visual input to compensate for poor proprioception and balance, with extra attention required to stand, walk, and use walking aids.

Walking with Robotics

Robotic systems fall into the following categories: (1) treadmill robotics, (2) foot-plate robotics, (3) overground robotics, (4) active foot orthoses, and (5) stationary gait and ankle trainers.[53] Swinnen and colleagues[54] assessed the effectiveness of RAST using a treadmill robot (Lokomat, Hocomo, Zurich, Switzerland) in patients with SCI. Walking ability and performance were measured, and no evidence was found that RAST improves walking function more than other training strategies. Field Fote and Roach[52] published a well-designed study comparing RAST with treadmill and overground training, with and without electrical stimulation. After training for 5 days per week for 12 weeks, the walking speed improved with either overground or treadmill training with stimulation and with treadmill training with manual assistance. Walking distance improved to a greater extent with overground training with stimulation.[52] RAST may require active participation of patients for walking gains; in fact, the metabolic cost was low during RAST with passive walking.[55] RAST, thus, requires active walking to increase cardiopulmonary fitness in those with SCI.

Other methods of RAST include an electromechanical gait trainer, active and passive exoskeletons, and hybrid systems. The electromechanical gait trainer uses moving plates to simulate the walking stance and swing phases.[56] This simulation produces similar results to training with manual assistance, but older and frailer patients participated at a lower rate. This device is marketed with FES capabilities (Gait Trainer GT1, Reha-Stim, Berlin, Germany). One motorized robotic exoskeleton enables unassisted walking and is approved by the Food and Drug Administration (FDA) for use in clinical settings (ReWalk, Argo Medical, Israel). During feasibility trials, 10 patients with thoracic motor complete SCI used this device to complete a 6MWT to measure walking endurance. They walked for 11 to 150 m, although there was a high variability between patients.[57] Two patients were unable to clear the foot during swing causing short strides, thus the device is not appropriate for all patients. A second robotic walking device is in clinical trials and is derived from the eLegs device originally designed by Berkeley Bionics (Ekso, Ekso Bionics, Richmond, California) and currently has FDA approval for use in a hospital setting. Lastly, there is a wearable robotic assistive device that augments walking via robotic hip and knee flexion and extension but is only available for rental in Japan (HAL, Cyberdyne, Tsukuba, Japan).

Walking with Resistance and Proprioception

Proprioceptive feedback and anticipatory motor commands contribute to adaptive strategies as shown when resistance is added to the leg during walking.[58,59] Lower extremity flexor activity is enhanced when loading the legs during the swing phase with weights or robotic-applied velocity-dependent resistance in patients with iSCI.[58] Knee flexor activity increased consistently, whereas hip and ankle flexor activity increased less consistently during the swing phase. Directly after the resistance was removed, knee flexion activity remained enhanced. Houldin and colleagues[59] showed that individuals with iSCI modulate flexor muscle activity similarly to uninjured controls. All patients increased rectus femoris activity during swing, and those with iSCI showed weak modulation of muscle activity to different resistance levels. Directly after the resistance was removed, the controls responded with a high step, whereas those with iSCI increased step length. The aftereffect size was related to the resistance level, but those with SCI exhibited a negative relationship between the aftereffect size and locomotor function. This finding signified that those with iSCI can form anticipatory motor commands.

Skill Training

Skill training uses overground walking that is intensive, variable, and relevant to daily walking. This training may facilitate transfer of gains to activities of daily living, household or community ambulation.[60] Negotiating curbs, doors, and uneven terrain is important to patients with limited ambulation. The effectiveness of skill training was determined in 4 participants with iSCI and compared with BWSTT. Skill training was based on 3 principles: (1) tasks practiced were important for daily walking, (2) a variety of environments and conditions were used to simulate daily life, and (3) tasks practiced were sufficiently challenging to induce errors. The third principle was essential because learning is augmented in situations whereby errors are induced rather than suppressed. The minimal clinically important difference for walking speed was 0.05 m/s or more. Walking speed improvements either met or exceeded this value, especially with skill training; the median speed improvement was 0.09 m/s for skill training and 0.01 m/s for BWSTT. Endurance, obstacle clearance, and stair climbing also improved. Three patients retained their speed gains after 3 months.

The Role of FES in Improving Walking Ability

FES can enhance function, improve muscle strength, and increase cardiorespiratory fitness; but small sample sizes and lack of generalizability limit the extrapolation of these benefits to the wider population.[12,61] A neuroprosthesis with FES facilitates walking and exercise,[62–64] and bracing with FES provides additional benefits in some patients.[65,66] Stimulation can be delivered via surface electrodes or implanted systems with intramuscular electrodes. In the near future, implanted peripheral nerve arrays and intraspinal microstimulation will deliver stimulation for walking. Although implanted systems require surgery, invasive procedures can be as acceptable as less invasive therapy.[67] The advantages of neuroprostheses are detailed in the review by Mushahwar and colleagues.[63] Surface FES devices, such as the Odstock (Odstock Medical Limited, Salisbury, Wiltshire, UK) and Parastep (Sigmedics, Inc, Fairborn, OH) devices, enable walking and may also facilitate exercise.[68] Patients with thoracic-level spinal cord injuries can stand and ambulate short distances with FES but with a high degree of performance variability across individuals. The factors that influence this variability have yet to be identified.

The benefits of FES walking are dependent on the nature of the injury. Although there are concerns about the lack of functionality of FES as an intervention,[61] functional improvement has been demonstrated with surface and implanted FES systems.[62,64,68,69] These systems produce therapeutic and functional gains. An implanted neuroprosthesis can maximize walking function in iSCI, as shown in 2 case studies.[62,64] After BWSTT and 12 weeks of training with a neuroprosthesis, the research participant remained nonambulatory[62]; but the neuroprosthesis maximal walking distance increased dramatically over 12 weeks, whereas the physiologic effort decreased. Moreover, the system was well tolerated, reliable, and allowed limited community ambulation where no ambulation existed before. Because the benefits and functionality are dependent on each patient's injury, FES has not been widely used in clinical practice. For instance, few patients with SCI used FES (2%), whereas 4 times more walked with an orthosis.[70] Most orthosis users had independent walking ability; but of those who used an FES system for walking, more than half had no functional walking ability.

FES can have carryover effects, suggesting that it is neurotherapeutic.[64,71] After training one patient for 12 weeks with an implanted iSCI FES walking system, volitional improvements were discovered in the 6-minute walking speed and distance, speed during the maximum distance walk, double support time, and 10-m walking speed.[64] Additional improvements were found when comparing post-training volitional and FES-assisted walking. FES-assisted gait improved with regard to maximum walking distance, peak knee flexion in swing, peak ankle dorsiflexion in swing, and knee extension moment. These achievements were sufficient to enable a change from household to limited community ambulation. The patient could also perform multiple walks per day with FES, although this was impossible volitionally. Similar outcomes were reported in patients with iSCI who were ambulatory before FES treatment, including an increase in voluntary strength, a decrease in energy cost, an increase in maximum walking distance, speed and step length, and improved joint kinematics.[71]

Muscle strength plays a role in determining whether to give high-functioning patients with iSCI a hinged ankle foot orthosis (AFO) or FES.[65] Patients with weaker hip flexors, knee flexors, and ankle dorsiflexors showed the greatest increases in walking speed with FES. Using an AFO and FES together increased foot clearance during swing and increased walking speed and endurance over using each device individually. When used alone, both increased walking speed and endurance, whereas foot clearance only improved with FES.

Fatigability of electrically stimulated paralyzed muscles can limit the use of FES for walking[72] and is related to factors including muscle atrophy and decreased cardiovascular capacity. The muscles are also activated nonphysiologically by FES with fast twitch fibers recruited first. For those with complete SCI who use FES, time to muscle fatigue can hamper walking, but progressive interval training with FES can improve time to muscle fatigue.[73] This progressive interval training with FES was effective for strength and endurance improvements in the large lower leg muscles. All participants increased the time to muscle fatigue during walking, but the total walking distance increased modestly for some and markedly for others (up to 300%). This intersubject variability was also seen in the progressive improvement over the training period.

Hybrid neuroprostheses for those with a complete SCI can restore more normal walking mechanics, such as stance phase knee flexion and hip coupling, using a combination of lower extremity bracing plus FES.[66,74–76] The experimental system included a novel hip reciprocating mechanism that allowed each hip to automatically lock or rotate freely for walking or stair climbing.[66,74] This mechanism provided smooth control at the hip with increased hip flexion compared with an isocentric reciprocating gait orthosis.[74] It has been used successfully with 2 knee mechanisms: a stance control knee that automatically locks during stance to support the body weight and prevent knee collapse[76] and a variable impedance knee that prevents knee collapse while allowing controlled knee flexion.[75] This mechanism also offsets fatigue during walking and allows walking over uneven ground and stair descent.

CHALLENGES TO WALKING AFTER SCI

Innovative inpatient and postdischarge strategies are needed to address the challenges of walking for individuals with SCI.[8] These strategies include psychological support and self-help mental health strategies. Challenges to walking range from negotiating curbs, donning and doffing braces or a surface FES system, FES surgical implantation, fear of falling, and muscle fatigue. Fear of falling can restrict rehabilitation, curtail the walking time after discharge, and influence postural control in those who walk with orthoses and crutches.[37] Community walking can be challenging, but clearing obstacles and climbing stairs can be improved with training.[60] Those with iSCI adopt different movement strategies when faced with walking over obstacles partly because of limited hip flexion.[77] Prescription medication use can also be a barrier to walking. In one study, the distances covered under medication were more likely to be limited to less than 150 ft, with medication use inversely related to achieving community ambulation distances of more than 1000 ft.[78]

REFERENCES

1. Morse LR, Stolzmann K, Nguyen HP, et al. Association between mobility mode and C-reactive protein levels in men with chronic spinal cord injury. Arch Phys Med Rehabil 2008;89:726–31.
2. Behrman AL, Harkema SJ. Physical rehabilitation as an agent for recovery after spinal cord injury. Phys Med Rehabil Clin N Am 2007;18:183–202.
3. Findikoglu G, Gunduz B, Uzun H, et al. Investigation of cartilage degradation in patients with spinal cord injury by CTX-II. Spinal Cord 2012;50:136–40.
4. Biering-Sorensen F, Hansen B, Lee BS. Non-pharmacological treatment and prevention of bone loss after spinal cord injury: a systematic review. Spinal Cord 2009;47(7):508–18.
5. Morse LR, Sudhakar S, Danilack V, et al. Association between sclerostin and bone density in chronic spinal cord injury. J Bone Miner Res 2012;27:352–9.
6. Lichy AM, Groah S. Asymmetric lower-limb bone loss after spinal cord injury: case report. J Rehabil Res Dev 2012;49(2):221–6.
7. Riggins MS, Kankipati P, Oyster ML, et al. The relationship between quality of life and change in mobility 1 year postinjury in individuals with spinal cord injury. Arch Phys Med Rehabil 2011;92:1027–33.
8. Jannings W, Pryor J. The experiences and needs of persons with spinal cord injury who can walk. Disabil Rehabil 2012;34:1820–6.
9. Harvey LA, Adams R, Chu J, et al. A comparison of patients' and physiotherapists' expectations about walking post spinal cord injury: a longitudinal cohort study. Spinal Cord 2012;50(7):548–52.
10. Patrick JH. Case for gait analysis as part of the management of incomplete spinal cord injury. Spinal Cord 2003;41:479–82.
11. van Middendorp JJ, Hosman AJ, Pouw MH, et al. ASIA impairment scale conversion in traumatic SCI: is it related with the ability to walk? A descriptive

comparison with functional ambulation outcome measures in 273 patients. Spinal Cord 2009;47:555–60.

12. Ditunno J, Scivoletto G. Clinical relevance of gait research applied to clinical trials in spinal cord injury. Brain Res Bull 2009;78:35–42.

13. Slavin MD, Kisala PA, Jette AM, et al. Developing a contemporary functional outcome measure for spinal cord injury research. Spinal Cord 2010;48:262–7.

14. Kirschblum SC, Burns SP, Biering-Sorenson F. International standards for neurological classification of spinal cord injury (revised 2011). J Spinal Cord Med 2011; 34(6):535–46.

15. Ditunno JF. Outcome measures: evolution in clinical trials of neurological/functional recovery in spinal cord injury. Spinal Cord 2010;48:674–84.

16. Musselman K, Brunton K, Lam T, et al. Spinal cord injury functional ambulation profile: a new measure of walking ability. Neurorehabil Neural Repair 2011;25: 285–93.

17. Lam T, Noonan VK, Eng JJ. A systematic review of functional ambulation outcome measures in spinal cord injury. Spinal Cord 2008;46:246–54.

18. Furlan JC, Noonan V, Singh A, et al. Assessment of disability in patients with acute traumatic spinal cord injury: a systematic review of the literature. J Neurotrauma 2011;28:1413–30.

19. van Hedel HJ, Dietz V. Walking during daily life can be validly and responsively assessed in subjects with a spinal cord injury. Neurorehabil Neural Repair 2009;23:117–24.

20. Burns AS, Delparte JJ, Patrick M, et al. The reproducibility and convergent validity of the walking index for spinal cord injury (WISCI) in chronic spinal cord injury. Neurorehabil Neural Repair 2011;25:149–57.

21. Ditunno JF Jr, Burns AS, Marino RJ. Neurological and functional capacity outcome measures: essential to spinal cord injury clinical trials. J Rehabil Res Dev 2005;42:35–41.

22. Jackson AB, Carnel CT, Ditunno JF, et al. Outcome measures for gait and ambulation in the spinal cord injury population. J Spinal Cord Med 2008;31:487–99.

23. van Hedel HJ, Wirz M, Dietz V. Standardized assessment of walking capacity after spinal cord injury: the European network approach. Neurol Res 2008;30:61–73.

24. van Hedel HJ, Wirz M, Dietz V. Assessing walking ability in subjects with spinal cord injury: validity and reliability of 3 walking tests. Arch Phys Med Rehabil 2005;86:190–6.

25. van Hedel HJ, Dietz V. Rehabilitation of locomotion after spinal cord injury. Restor Neurol Neurosci 2010;28:123–34.

26. Zörner B, Blanckenhorn WU, Dietz V, et al. Clinical algorithm for improved prediction of ambulation and patient stratification after incomplete spinal cord injury. J Neurotrauma 2010;27:241–52.

27. Yang JF, Norton J, Nevett-Duchcherer J, et al. Volitional muscle strength in the legs predicts changes in walking speed following locomotor training in people with chronic spinal cord injury. Phys Ther 2011;91:931–43.

28. Crozier KS, Cheng LL, Graziani V, et al. Spinal cord injury: prognosis for ambulation based on quadriceps recovery. Paraplegia 1992;30:762–7.

29. Scivoletto G, Cosentino E, Mammone A, et al. Inflammatory myelopathies and traumatic spinal cord lesions: comparison of functional and neurological outcomes. Phys Ther 2008;88:471–84.

30. Kay E, Deutsch A, Chen D, et al. Effects of etiology on inpatient rehabilitation outcomes in 65- to 74-year-old patients with incomplete paraplegia from a nontraumatic spinal cord injury. PM R 2010;2(6):504–13.

31. New PW. Functional outcomes and disability after nontraumatic spinal cord injury rehabilitation: results from a retrospective study. Arch Phys Med Rehabil 2005;86: 250–61.
32. New PW, Epi MC. Influence of age and gender on rehabilitation outcomes in non-traumatic spinal cord injury. J Spinal Cord Med 2007;30:225–37.
33. Gorgey AS, Poarch H, Miller J, et al. Locomotor and resistance training restore walking in an elderly person with a chronic incomplete spinal cord injury. Neuro-Rehabilitation 2010;26:127–33.
34. Krause J, Carter RE, Brotherton S. Association of mode of locomotion and inde-pendence in locomotion with long-term outcomes after spinal cord injury. J Spinal Cord Med 2009;32:237–48.
35. Jain NB, Higgins LD, Katz JN, et al. Association of shoulder pain with the use of mobility devices in persons with chronic spinal cord injury. PM R 2010;2:896–900.
36. Brotherton SS, Krause JS, Nietert PJ. A pilot study of factors associated with falls in individuals with incomplete spinal cord injury. J Spinal Cord Med 2007;30: 243–50.
37. John LT, Cherian B, Babu A. Postural control and fear of falling in persons with low-level paraplegia. J Rehabil Res Dev 2010;47:497–502.
38. Nadeau S, Duclos C, Bouyer L, et al. Guiding task-oriented gait training after stroke or spinal cord injury by means of a biomechanical gait analysis. Prog Brain Res 2011;192:161–80.
39. Krawetz P, Nance P. Gait analysis of spinal cord injured subjects: effects of injury level and spasticity. Arch Phys Med Rehabil 1996;77:635–8.
40. Gil-Agudo A, Pérez-Nombela S, Forner-Cordero A, et al. Gait kinematic analysis in patients with a mild form of central cord syndrome. J Neuroeng Rehabil 2011;8: 7–16.
41. Dobkin BH, Apple D, Barbeau H, et al. Methods for a randomized trial of weight-supported treadmill training versus conventional training for walking during inpa-tient rehabilitation after incomplete traumatic spinal cord injury. Neurorehabil Neural Repair 2003;17:153–67.
42. Dobkin B, Barbeau H, Deforge D, et al. The evolution of walking-related outcomes over the first 12 weeks of rehabilitation for incomplete traumatic spinal cord injury: the multicenter randomized Spinal Cord Injury Locomotor Trial. Neurorehabil Neural Repair 2007;21:25–35.
43. Dobkin BH, Duncan P. Should body weight-supported treadmill training and robotic assistive steppers for locomotor training trot back to the starting gate? Neurorehabil Neural Repair 2012;46(4):308–17.
44. Mehrholz J, Kugler J, Pohl M. Locomotor training for walking after spinal cord injury. Cochrane Database Syst Rev 2008;(2):CD006676.
45. Alexeeva N, Sames C, Jacobs PL, et al. Comparison of training methods to improve walking in persons with chronic spinal cord injury: a randomized clinical trial. J Spinal Cord Med 2011;34:362–79.
46. Chen XY, Chen Y, Wang Y, et al. Reflex conditioning: a new strategy for improving motor function after spinal cord injury. Ann N Y Acad Sci 2010;1198(Suppl 1): E12–21.
47. Knikou M, Angeli CA, Ferreira CK, et al. Soleus H-reflex modulation during body weight support treadmill walking in spinal cord intact and injured subjects. Exp Brain Res 2009;193:397–407.
48. Benito Penalva J, Opisso E, Medina J, et al. H reflex modulation by transcranial magnetic stimulation in spinal cord injury subjects after gait training with electro-mechanical systems. Spinal Cord 2010;48:400–6.

49. Barbeau H, Norman K, Fung J, et al. Does neurorehabilitation play a role in the recovery of walking in neurological populations? Ann N Y Acad Sci 1998;860: 377–92.
50. Field-Fote EC. Spinal cord control of movement: implications for locomotor rehabilitation following spinal cord injury. Phys Ther 2000;80:477–84.
51. Hicks AL, Ginis KA. Treadmill training after spinal cord injury: it's not just about the walking. J Rehabil Res Dev 2008;45:241–8.
52. Field-Fote EC, Roach KE. Influence of a locomotor training approach on walking speed and distance in people with chronic spinal cord injury: a randomized clinical trial. Phys Ther 2011;91:48–60.
53. Diaz I, Gil JJ, Sanchez E. Lower-limb robotic rehabilitation: literature review and challenges. J Robotics 2011;2011:1–11.
54. Swinnen E, Duerinck S, Baeyens JP, et al. Effectiveness of robot-assisted gait training in persons with spinal cord injury: a systematic review. J Rehabil Med 2010;42:520–6.
55. Jack LP, Purcell M, Allan DB, et al. The metabolic cost of passive walking during robotics-assisted treadmill exercise. Technol Health Care 2011;19:21–7.
56. Hesse S, Werner C. Connecting research to the needs of patients and clinicians. Brain Res Bull 2009;78:26–34.
57. Esquenazi A, Coulter T, Packel A, et al. Safety and performance of ReWalk reciprocating gait orthosis. PM R 2010;2(9):S158–9.
58. Lam T, Wirz M, Lünenburger L, et al. Swing phase resistance enhances flexor muscle activity during treadmill locomotion in incomplete spinal cord injury. Neurorehabil Neural Repair 2008;22:438–46.
59. Houldin A, Luttin K, Lam T. Locomotor adaptations and aftereffects to resistance during walking in individuals with spinal cord injury. J Neurophysiol 2011;106: 247–58.
60. Musselman KE, Fouad K, Misiaszek JE, et al. Training of walking skills overground and on the treadmill: case series on individuals with incomplete spinal cord injury. Phys Ther 2009;89:601–11.
61. Nightingale EJ, Raymond J, Middleton JW, et al. Benefits of FES gait in a spinal cord injured population. Spinal Cord 2007;45:646–57.
62. Hardin E, Kobetic R, Murray L, et al. Walking after incomplete spinal cord injury using an implanted FES system: a case report. J Rehabil Res Dev 2007;44:333–46.
63. Mushahwar VK, Jacobs PL, Normann RA, et al. New functional electrical stimulation approaches to standing and walking. J Neural Eng 2007;4:S181–97.
64. Bailey SN, Hardin EC, Kobetic R, et al. Neurotherapeutic and neuroprosthetic effects of implanted functional electrical stimulation for ambulation after incomplete spinal cord injury. J Rehabil Res Dev 2010;47:7–16.
65. Kim CM, Eng JJ, Whittaker MW. Effects of a simple functional electric system and/ or a hinged ankle-foot orthosis on walking in persons with incomplete spinal cord injury. Arch Phys Med Rehabil 2004;85:1718–23.
66. Kobetic R, To CS, Schnellenberger JR, et al. Development of hybrid orthosis for standing, walking, and stair climbing after spinal cord injury. J Rehabil Res Dev 2009;46(3):447–62.
67. Brown-Triolo DL, Roach MJ, Nelson K, et al. Consumer perspectives on mobility: implications for neuroprosthesis design. J Rehabil Res Dev 2002;39(6):659–69.
68. Klose KJ, Jacobs PL, Broton JG, et al. Evaluation of a training program for persons with SCI paraplegia using the Parastep 1 ambulation system: part 1. Ambulation performance and anthropometric measures. Arch Phys Med Rehabil 1997;78:789–93.

69. Dutta A, Kobetic R, Triolo RJ. Walking after partial paralysis assisted with EMG-triggered or switch-triggered functional electrical stimulation—two case studies. IEEE Int Conf Rehabil Robot 2011;2011:5975383.
70. Maxwell DJ, Granat MH, Baardman G, et al. Demand for and use of functional electrical stimulation systems and conventional orthoses in the spinal lesioned community of the UK. Artif Organs 1999;23:410–2.
71. Johnston TE, Finson RL, Smith BT, et al. Functional electrical stimulation for augmented walking in adolescents with incomplete spinal cord injury. J Spinal Cord Med 2003;26:390–400.
72. Glaser RM. Physiologic aspects of spinal cord injury and functional neuromuscular stimulation. Cent Nerv Syst Trauma 1986;3:49–62.
73. Crosbie J, Russold M, Raymond J, et al. Functional electrical stimulation-supported interval training following sensorimotor-complete spinal cord injury: a case series. Neuromodulation 2009;12:224–31.
74. Audu ML, To CS, Kobetic R, et al. Gait evaluation of a novel hip constraint orthosis with implication for walking in paraplegia. IEEE Trans Neural Syst Rehabil Eng 2010;18(6):610–8.
75. Bulea TC, Kobetic R, Triolo RJ. Restoration of stance phase knee flexion during walking after spinal cord injury using a variable impedance orthosis. Conf Proc IEEE Eng Med Biol Soc 2011;2011:608–11.
76. To CS, Kobetic R, Bulea TC, et al. Stance control knee mechanism for lower-limb support in hybrid neuroprosthesis. J Rehabil Res Dev 2011;48(7):839–50.
77. Ladouceur M, Barbeau H, McFadyen BJ. Kinematic adaptations of spinal cord-injured subjects during obstructed walking. Neurorehabil Neural Repair 2003;17:25–31.
78. Kohout RK, Saunders LL, Krause JS. The relationship between prescription medication use and ability to ambulate distances after spinal cord injury. Arch Phys Med Rehabil 2011;92:1246–9.

Ambulation and Parkinson Disease

Shinichi Amano, BS, Ryan T. Roemmich, BS, Jared W. Skinner, MS,
Chris J. Hass, PhD*

KEYWORDS

- Parkinson disease • Basal ganglia • Pedunculopontine nucleus • Postural instability
- Gait disturbance • Biomechanics • Rehabilitation • Deep brain stimulation

KEY POINTS

- Parkinson disease (PD) is characterized pathologically by the presence of nigrostriatal dopaminergic cell loss in the basal ganglia, resulting in both motor and nonmotor symptoms. The cardinal features of PD include resting tremor, rigidity, akinesia/bradykinesia, and postural instability and gait disturbance (PIGD).
- In addition to basal ganglia disturbance, it has been suggested that activity of the cerebellum and pedunculopontine nucleus is also altered in persons with PD. Given that both brain areas contribute to locomotor control, gait disturbance in persons with PD seems to manifest as a result of abnormal activity within a variety of neural components.
- PIGD is a particularly debilitating motor feature of persons with PD, leading to the findings that more than 70% of persons with PD fall during the course of their disease, often resulting in fractures.
- Parkinsonian gait is characterized by bradykinesia, stooped posture, high stride-to-stride variability, and, in some persons, freezing episodes. Persons with PD also have decreased stability during both static and dynamic motor tasks.
- Although various treatment methods (pharmacologic, surgical, and physical therapy based) have been suggested to alleviate PIGD symptoms with varying degrees of effectiveness, further investigations should pool insights obtained from neurologic, physiologic, and biomechanical perspectives to advance understanding of PIGD in persons with PD and develop effective interventions that specifically address these deficits.

INTRODUCTION

Parkinson disease (PD) is a chronic and progressive neurodegenerative disorder that leads to a wide variety of both motor and nonmotor features. PD is characterized pathologically by the presence of nigrostriatal dopaminergic cell loss in the basal ganglia.

Disclosures: Nil.
Conflict of interest: Nil.
Department of Applied Physiology and Kinesiology, College of Health and Human Performance, University of Florida, Room 100, FLG, PO Box 118205, Gainesville, FL 32611, USA
* Corresponding author.
E-mail address: cjhass@hhp.ufl.edu

Phys Med Rehabil Clin N Am 24 (2013) 371–392
http://dx.doi.org/10.1016/j.pmr.2012.11.003
1047-9651/13/$ – see front matter © 2013 Elsevier Inc. All rights reserved.

pmr.theclinics.com

The cardinal symptoms of PD include resting tremor, rigidity, akinesia/bradykinesia, and postural instability and gait disturbance (PIGD). Of these cardinal motor features, PIGD is one of the most disabling,[1,2] leading to not only decreased mobility and increased fall frequency but also reduction in quality of life. It is estimated that more than 70% of persons with PD fall during the course of their disease, often resulting in fractures.[2–5] Physical inactivity as a consequence of frequent falls or fear of falling can also substantially shorten life expectancy for persons with PD.[2] To improve the quality of life for persons with PD, many research studies have evaluated the underlying mechanisms that cause PIGD and have focused on the evaluation of intervention strategies designed to reverse or alleviate PIGD in this population.

This article reviews (1) the neuropathology affecting PIGD in persons with PD, (2) the behavioral manifestation of PIGD, and (3) currently available surgical, pharmacologic, and physical therapy-based interventions to combat PIGD.

NEUROPATHOLOGY OF PIGD IN PARKINSON DISEASE

As a result of research spanning several decades, the neuropathology of parkinsonian motor features and their relationships to dysfunction of the basal ganglia and other subcortical structures are becoming increasingly well understood. The basal ganglia are a multifunctional group of subcortical nuclei (the striatum, pallidum, subthalamic nucleus [STN], and substantia nigra) that maintain a vast series of inputs and outputs to transmit signals throughout the brain (**Fig. 1**). The basal ganglia interact largely with other cerebral motor structures, including the cortex, midbrain, thalamus, and cerebellum, to execute and coordinate voluntary movements such as gait. Pivotal research in the 1980s significantly advanced the understanding of basal ganglia circuitry, outlining not only connections within subcortical structures but also interactions between the basal ganglia and multiple areas of the cortex. Alexander and colleagues[6]

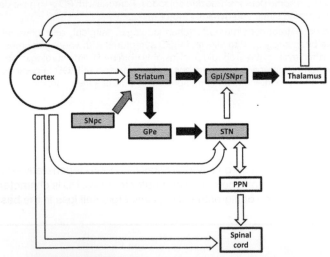

Fig. 1. Basic circuitry of the basal ganglia and related structures. (*Black arrows*) Inhibitory GABAergic transmissions; (*white arrows*) excitatory glutamatergic (or, in the case of PPN, cholinergic) transmissions; (*gray arrows*) dopaminergic transmissions; (*gray boxes*) nuclei intrinsic to the basal ganglia. The striatum is composed of the putamen and the caudate nucleus. GABA, γ-aminobutyric acid; GPe, globus pallidus externus; GPi, globus pallidus internus; PPN, pedunculopontine nucleus; SNpc, substantia nigra pars compacta; SNpr, substantia nigra pars reticulata.

expanded on traditional views that proposed that basal ganglia output primarily consisted of connections to the primary motor cortex,[7,8] and they were among the first to suggest the organization of functionally distinct basal ganglia circuitry, postulating connections between the basal ganglia and multiple cortical areas controlling various functions. For instance, basal ganglia connections with the premotor areas and primary motor and somatosensory cortices are influential on motor function, whereas interactions with structures within the prefrontal cortex and the anterior cingulate are important for cognition.

The ideology of functional segregation of interactions between the basal ganglia and cortical structures eventually led to the identification of 3 primary pathways through which the basal ganglia, thalamus, and cortex interact: the hyperdirect, direct, and indirect pathways.[9–11] When voluntarily initiating movement, these 3 pathways are essential in coordinating the movement through a highly specific selection of available motor programs.[12] First, the hyperdirect pathway is thought to reset the system by suppressing both intended and competing actions by inhibiting activity of the motor cortex.[13] The direct pathway subsequently facilitates the desired motor program for execution of the selected action by exciting the cortex.[11,14] The indirect pathway then inhibits competing motor programs to efficiently execute the desired movement.[15]

In persons with PD, degeneration of dopaminergic neurons within the pars compacta of the substantia nigra disrupts the normal function of motor program selection by the basal ganglia circuitry,[16,17] resulting in improper enhancement of desired motor programs and faulty inhibition of competing programs. These irregularities in PD motor control manifest in gait patterns that are characterized by rigidity, bradykinesia, and postural instability[18] (discussed later). Dopaminergic dysfunction often has devastating consequences on gait, because locomotion is influenced not only directly by the aforementioned basal ganglia interactions with the thalamus and cortex but also, perhaps predominantly, through reciprocal circuitry connecting the basal ganglia and the midbrain locomotor region (MLR).[19,20] In addition to basal ganglia structures, the pedunculopontine nucleus (PPN) of the MLR has recently become a primary target for treatments designed to achieve locomotor improvement.[21,22]

The PPN is composed primarily of cholinergic neurons, which have been shown to be reduced in some persons with PD,[23] particularly those who experience frequent falling and balance deficits.[24] Like the basal ganglia, the PPN seems to have connections to various motor regions throughout the central nervous system. In addition to reciprocal connections with the basal ganglia, the PPN also interacts with important locomotor control regions in the cerebellum[25] and the spinal cord[26,27] to influence the initiation, speed manipulation, and termination of gait.[19] Further, recent research on these interactions has produced intriguing results that suggest that dysfunction of the PPN may be a major contributor to the freezing of gait (FOG) phenomenon frequently observed in persons with PD.[28,29] The effects of PPN stimulation on FOG have become a highly emphasized area of research in the treatment of parkinsonian locomotor deficits.[30–33]

Because the cerebellum is theorized to share connections with both the thalamus and the PPN, abnormal cerebellar function has been suggested to also contribute to some of the locomotor changes that occur in persons with PD. Hyperactivity of the cerebellum has been observed in persons with PD when performing upper extremity movements[34–36] and walking.[37] This cerebellar hyperactivity may act to influence cortical mechanisms as necessary compensation for motor control dysfunction of the basal ganglia. However, this abnormal cerebellar function may limit adaptability of gait in PD, because Jayaram and colleagues[38] recently observed that cerebellar depression is proportional to the ability to learn and store different gait patterns. Thus, altered cerebellar function in PD may have important effects on transitional periods during gait in which the rhythmicity and timing must be manipulated to safely and efficiently adapt locomotor patterns. In this way, PIGD in persons with PD seems to be manifested as a multifactorial motor complication involving cortical, subcortical, and cerebellar structures of the brain.

PIGD IN PARKINSON DISEASE

PIGD is one of the most debilitating symptoms of PD, characterized by spatial and temporal disturbances compared with neurologically healthy adults.[39] Gait disturbances in PD are divided into 2 types: episodic and continuous (**Table 1**).[39] Episodic gait disturbances (see **Table 1**) occur infrequently and abruptly, in an apparently random manner.[2,40] These include festination, hesitation of gait, and FOG.[41] In contrast, continuous gait disturbances (see **Table 1**) are persistent and apparent throughout the waking day.[42] For instance, parkinsonian gait is hypokinetic; characterized by decreased gait

Table 1
Characteristics of PIGDs in Parkinson disease

Gait Disturbances	Manifestation of PIGD
Episodic	
(1) Gait initiation	Decreased COM-COP displacement
	Increased variability in initial step length
	Decreased dynamic postural support
	Decreased mobility
	Reduced BOS
	Increased risk of falling
(2) Festination	Reduced stride length
	Increased cadence
	Decreased gait velocity
	Increased risk of falling
	Decreased COG-BOS displacement
(3) Gait termination	Decreased gait velocity before termination
	Increased cadence before termination
	Abnormal muscle activation
	Decreased dynamic postural support
	Increased risk of falling
(4) Freezing of gait	Commonly occurring in advanced stage
	Decreased mobility
	Decreased dynamic postural support
	Increased risk of falling
Continuous	
(1) Gait	Decreased gait velocity, stride length, and time without change in cadence
	Inability to modulate stride length
	Decreased arm swing
	Increased double support time
	Decreased dynamic postural support
	Decreased bilateral coordinated gait patterns
	Increased asymmetry (early stages)
	Increased gait variability
	Increased risk of falling

Abbreviations: BOS, base of support; COG, center of gravity; COM, center of mass; COP, center of pressure.

velocity with short, slow steps[18,43]; slowed and decreased arm swing[44]; increased double-limb support[45,46]; and decreased dynamic postural stability.[46–48] In persons with PD, there is a decreased ability to internally control the center of mass (COM) during self-directed activities such as initiating gait, turning, and stopping, and this inability is commonly associated with falls.[45,49,50] Each task involves control of the COM whether in response to unexpected perturbations or to planned transitions between 2 stable postures.[51,52] This inability to self-regulate postural changes manifests in deficits observed in gait initiation (GI) and gait termination.

GI

GI is a functional task that requires a voluntary shift in the center of pressure (COP) from a 2-leg stance into an alternating single-leg stance, thus temporarily reducing the person's base of support (BOS) (see **Table 1**).[50,51,53] These voluntary postural shifts, known as anticipatory postural adjustments (APAs), help generate the momentum needed to initiate forward motion while maintaining balance.[50,51,53] Persons with PD have a deficit in maintaining postural stability during the transitional stages between states of static and dynamic equilibrium, such as during GI, gait termination, or turning.[49–51,53] The increased difficulty in initiating gait may stem from episodes of start hesitation, which are frequently observed in persons with PD and can occur while on and off dopaminergic medication.[54] GI requires a controlled muscular effort to decouple the body's COM from the COP to generate forward motion.[51,55,56] Patterns of abnormal electromyographic (EMG) activity in the lower extremities has been observed in persons with PD, including cocontraction of agonist and antagonist muscles,[57] increased variability in motor unit recruitment,[58,59] and decreased frequency and magnitude in first agonist burst.[59] These EMG abnormalities likely stem from deficits in the corticospinal activation of the muscle.[60] Control of the COM and COP during GI has major implications for momentum generation and balance control.[51,56] The increased displacement of the COM from the COP generates a larger moment arm for the ground reaction forces to drive momentum generation.[51] The transition from double-limb support to an unstable single-limb support decreases dynamic stability by reducing the BOS.[50,51,53,55] During GI, limiting the COM-COP displacement observed in persons with PD seems to compensate for dynamic postural control.[51,53,56] Our previous study found that, when alternating foot position from the normal double-limb support stance during GI, persons with PD were able to initiate gait in a similar manner as their neurologically healthy peers.[61] These findings should be expanded to design effective intervention programs that address issues with postural stability during transitions from static and dynamic positions to minimize the risk of falling.

Gait

As mentioned earlier, persons with PD often walk with reduced gait speed, shorter stride length, reduced arm swing, and decreased postural stability (see **Table 1**). Reductions in gait velocity stem from diminished stride length in persons with PD, whereas cadence is typically unaffected.[45,62] Decreased stride length has been suggested as a compensatory strategy to maintain stability by limiting the displacement of the COM relative to the BOS.[63,64] Another strategy often implemented by persons with PD to increase dynamic stability is the unique parkinsonian disturbance known as festinating gait, which is characterized by rapid, hypometric steps that minimize displacement of center of gravity relative to the BOS and increase double-limb support time (see **Table 1**).[65] This compensatory gait mechanism is likely generated in response to the inability to control motor processes that simultaneously require regularity, rhythmicity, and symmetry in movements between limbs to create coordinated gait patterns.[66] Often, the ability to synchronize these processes bilaterally are disrupted in PD, resulting in increased gait asymmetry, diminished bilateral coordination, and high stride-to-stride variability.[39,66,67] Abnormal gait variability has been shown in all stages of the disease and seems to increase with disease severity.[39,58] Increased variability in PD locomotion is not limited to steady-state gait; data from our laboratory has shown that persons with PD also show increased variability in stepping during GI compared with their neurologically healthy peers.[43] Previous research has shown a robust relationship between increased variability in both gait and GI and falling in a multitude of healthy and pathologic populations, including PD.[54,68–70] Thus, abnormally high gait variability may also be a target for interventions to reduce falling in persons with PD.

Gait Termination

Gait termination is the transition from steady-state walking to a static stance and is a common motor task performed throughout the course of the waking day. Similar to GI, gait termination is achieved through a series of APAs that control the forward progression of the body and dissipate the kinetic energy generated by the forward momentum of walking to achieve a stable static position.[52,71] In PD, there is a decreased ability to modulate lower extremity muscular activity and ground reaction forces during gait termination (see **Table 1**).[72–74] Persons with PD have difficulty modulating the rate of force generation[52,73,74] because of impaired muscle activation indicated by abnormal EMG patterns.[59,75] This anomaly is also experienced during periods in which APAs are required to shift the COM in preparation for gait termination.[71] Gait termination involves interlimb coordination that results in an increase in deceleration forces in the leading limb and a consequential decrease in acceleration in the trailing limb.[52,55,71,76] When healthy adults rapidly terminate gait, a set of motor commands are sent to the muscle of the lead and trail limbs.[55,74,77] Persons with PD have difficulty switching from one set of motor commands to another. Compared with neurologically healthy age-matched peers, persons with PD are less able to modulate these forces and associated impulses when given an unexpected signal to stop. Given the potential risk of falls when terminating gait, it is imperative that intervention strategies be implemented using gait termination tasks to improve unplanned stopping and decrease the risk of falls.

Falling

Persons with PD have an increased risk of falling compared with their neurologically healthy age-matched peers. Although approximately 30% of older adults fall at least once each year,[78] it has been suggested that this number rises to 70% in persons with PD.[79,80] Several prospective studies have shown that fall rates in persons with PD exceed those of healthy older adults,[64,79,80] and persons with PD are also at a significantly increased risk of suffering recurrent falls.[63,79] In response to an obvious need to address the mechanisms underlying falling in PD, multiple studies have established several predictors of future falls in persons with PD.[64,79,81,82] Previous falls and disease severity have been shown to be among the most reliable of these predictors of future falling. Generic fall-risk tests have been developed for the general elderly population, although it is uncertain whether these measures are equally sensitive for people with PD.[82] Therefore, there remains a need for research to identify predictors of first falls such that future research may focus on preventing falling before it starts in persons with PD.

FOG

One debilitating episodic phenomenon that occurs in some persons with PD is FOG, the involuntary and sudden cessation of gait that can occur during both the medically On and Off states (see **Table 1**).[2,45] Bilateral manifestation of FOG is common, but unilateral FOG may also occur, particularly in persons with asymmetrical parkinsonism or in the early stages of disease progression.[83] Duration of FOG episodes varies; some may last only a few seconds, whereas others may continue for 30 seconds or more.[66,84] FOG is often regarded as a feature of advanced PD and is commonly experienced during step initiation, transitioning through doorways, and turning.[45,85] FOG episodes have been strongly associated with decreased mobility and a greater loss of independence.[84] Gray and Hildebrand[47] reported that fall risk was increased among persons with FOG, and a strong correlation between falls and FOG has been observed in persons with PD.[79] Although the clinical significance of the relationship between falls and FOG in persons with PD has been well documented, the mechanisms underlying the FOG phenomenon remain an enigma. FOG episodes do not correlate with the cardinal features of parkinsonism such as tremor, bradykinesia, or rigidity,[45,84] and the pathophysiology leading to FOG in PD is a complex paradigm that is yet to be fully understood. Thus, it is crucial to implement appropriate intervention strategies to reduce FOG in persons with PD, because these interventions would likely minimize falling and improve quality of life.

PIGD deficits cumulatively contribute significantly to decreased mobility, loss of independence, and generally unstable movement patterns in persons with PD. Although PIGD deficits vary among individuals and are often highly task dependent (eg, gait, GI, gait termination, turning), most persons with PD are at least mildly affected by these debilitating motor symptoms. Because a wide variety of deficits regarding movement control and performance during these routine activities of daily living are frequently observed in PD, it is imperative to consider appropriate intervention strategies on a patient-specific basis.

INTERVENTION STRATEGIES ON PIGD FOR PERSONS WITH PARKINSON DISEASE

Because there is currently no cure for PD, treatment methods focus on minimizing, delaying, and alleviating motor deficits associated with PD. PIGD symptoms have become a primary target for various therapeutic techniques, because motor impairments have been strongly associated with declining quality of life in persons with PD.[86–88] A vast body of research into pharmacologic, surgical, and physical therapy–based interventions for PIGD in PD has accumulated over time, identifying treatment methods that target multiple motor deficits with varying degrees of effectiveness (**Table 2**).

Pharmacologic Intervention

The most common pharmacologic treatment used in PD is levodopa (see **Table 2**). Although levodopa has long been considered as the most effective medication to improve some motor features of PD, its effect on PIGD is controversial.[89] Previous studies investigating the effectiveness of levodopa on PIGD in PD have shown conflicting results. For instance, some studies have reported that gait velocity and stride length could be improved by levodopa; however, temporal gait parameters related to rhythm, such as stride duration and its variability, are typically not responsive to levodopa therapy.[62,90,91] Blin and colleagues[91] suggested that levodopa may be effective in enhancing activation of muscle groups responsible for gait, which may explain increased stride length and velocity. In contrast, ineffectiveness of levodopa therapy

Table 2
Summarized results of representative intervention strategy research

Intervention Type	Study (Investigators, Year)	N	Participants' Characteristics	Assessments	Significant PIGD Changes
Pharmacologic					
Levodopa	Blin et al,[91] 1991	20	Early to advanced stage (1–17 y after onset), H&Y scale: 1–4	Spatiotemporal and kinetic gait parameters: 1. Before L-dopa intake 2. After L-dopa intake	Gait velocity and stride length were increased after L-dopa intake (P<.05). Spatial and kinematic parameters (ie, stance duration, swing velocity, double support duration) also improved (P<.05). In contrast, temporal parameters (stride and swing duration, stride duration variability) were not improved
	Espay et al,[93] 2012	4	Moderate to advanced stage (6–20 y after onset), with a history of FOG in medicated state	Observation of FOG: 1. Medically Off state: after 1 h without medication 2. Medically On state: 45–60 min after intake of levodopa 3. Supra-on state	Medically On state FOG, which worsened in a dose-dependent fashion from the On to the Supra-on state, was observed Two patients also showed FOG during the Off state
Surgical					
(1) Traditional DBS (STN/GPi)	Rodriguez-Oroz et al,[111] 2005	69	Moderate to advanced stage (6–32 y after onset), H&Y scale: 2–5	UPDRS-III (assessed both On and Off medicated state): 1. Before DBS surgery 2. At 1 y after surgery 3. 3–4 y after surgery	Under medically Off state, total motor, gait, and postural stability scores in UPDRS were improved after 3–4 y after surgery (P<.0001), but these scores significantly worsened from 1 y after surgery (P<.002)

	Study	N	Stage	Comparison	Results
					Under medically On state, none of aforementioned scores improved after 3–4 y after surgery. Postural stability score significantly worsened ($P<.0001$)
(2) PPN-DBS	Stefani et al,[114] 2007	6	Advanced stage based on UPDRS motor score (>70)	UPDRS-III and UPDRS-III subscore (item 27–30) less than: 1. DBS-Off 2. PPN-DBS 3. STN-DBS 4. STN-DBS and PPN-DBS	Under medically Off condition, the UPDRS-III subscore (items 27–30) was significantly reduced by all 3 types of DBS (all $P<.01$), but PPN seemed more effective than STN alone. Under medically On condition, PPN-DBS ameliorated global UPDRS-III by 44% and STN-DBS and PPN-DBS improved by 66.4%. More importantly, UPDRS-III subscores (item 27–30) showed the benefit of STN-DBS and PPN-DBS ($P = .05$) and PPN-DBS (although n.s.) compared with STN-DBS
Physical Therapy					
(1) RT	Hass et al,[49] 2012	18	Mild to moderate stage (H&Y: 1–3)	GI testing: 1. 10-wk PRT 2. Control group	The PRT group showed improvements in the posterior displacement of the COP and the initial stride length and velocity during GI testing (all $P<.05$)

(continued on next page)

Table 2
(continued)

Intervention Type	Study (Investigators, Year)	N	Participants' Characteristics	Assessments	Significant PIGD Changes
(2) Tai chi	Hackney and Earhart,[142] 2008	33	Mild to moderate stage (H&Y:1.5–3)	UPDRS-III, BBS, TS, OLS, TUG, 6MW and forward/backward gait test: 1. 20 sessions of TC 2. Control group	TC significantly improved the BBS when compared with the Control (*P*<.05). However, forward walking and OLS did not improve in either group.
	Li et al,[141] 2012	195	Mild to severe stage (H&Y: 1–4)	LOS test, gait and strength test, functional-reach test, TUG, UPDRS-III, and number of falls: 1. 24 wk of TC 2. RT 3. Stretching	Overall, TC participants performed significantly better in LOS test, functional-reach test, and stride length in gait testing than those in the other 2 groups. Gait velocity, muscle strength, TUG, and UPDRS-III were significantly improved in both TC and RT groups compared with the stretching group. However, no significant difference was observed between TC and RT groups in these outcome measures
(3) TT	Herman et al,[147] 2007	9	Mild to moderate stage (H&Y: 1.5–3)	UPDRS-III, ABC, and spatiotemporal parameter during gait testing: 1. Before TT 2. 2–3 d after 6-wk TT 3. 4–5 wk after TT	UPDRS-III, gait velocity, and stride length were improved after 2–3 d after TT (all *P*<.05), and these benefits were maintained 4 wk after TT (all *P*<.05).

Abbreviations: BBS, Berg Balance Scale; DBS, deep brain stimulation; GPi, globus pallidus internus; H&Y, Hoehn and Yahr scale; LOS, limit of stability; 6MW, 6-minute-walk test; n.s., not significant; OLS, one-leg stance test; PRT, progressive resistance training; RT, resistance training; TC, tai chi; TS, tandem stance; TT, treadmill training; TUG, time-up-and-go test; UPDRS, Unified Parkinson Disease Rating Scale.

in improving gait variability may be caused by lack of force control during gait, which might indicate that PIGD also results from neurodegeneration within nondopaminergic pathways, possibly cholinergic pathways.[24,92]

The effects of dopaminergic therapy on FOG in PD are also controversial. Fahn[41] and the Parkinson Study Group reported that high doses of levodopa could delay or prevent the development of FOG in patients with early PD. In contrast, Espay and colleagues[93] reported medically On state FOG in patients with PD taking high doses. Thus, the results are conflicting and suggest that levodopa may successfully reduce FOG episodes in some persons with PD but also induce FOG in others if taken at higher doses. Overall, levodopa does not seem to be an effective option to ameliorate PIGD in patients with PD.

Surgical Interventions

Deep brain stimulation (DBS) is an alternative approach to alleviating a wide variety of parkinsonian motor features, including PIGD, tremor, rigidity, and hypokinesia.[94,95] DBS is an invasive surgical procedure during which a neurosurgeon implants an electrical lead directly into a target structure within the brain. The lead is connected through an extension wire to a battery-powered neurostimulator that is surgically implanted deep to the clavicle. Once the components are properly placed, the neurostimulator is activated to send electrical pulses to the lead(s) to alter the neuronal activity of the target brain structure and perhaps its downstream circuitry.

The most common locations of DBS implantation in persons with PD are the internal globus pallidus (GPi) and STN, because excessive neuronal activity in these areas has been suggested to cause cardinal motor symptoms of PD, such as tremor, bradykinesia, and rigidity (see **Table 2**).[96] This proposed rationale regarding the stimulation of GPi and STN was supported by nonhuman primate studies reporting improvement in motor function after lesion of these structures in parkinsonian animals and pallidotomy in persons with PD.[97–99] A previous study reported that STN and GPi stimulation significantly improved Unified Parkinson Disease Rating Scale (UPDRS) motor score, even after 2 years of treatment.[100] Regarding nonmotor PD symptoms, GPi stimulation seems to be effective in alleviating depression, whereas STN stimulation worsened the symptom. In contrast, STN-DBS could reduce the amount of medication usage compared with GPi-DBS. Because of the reported significant medication reduction in human cases[101] and effectiveness of STN lesion for the parkinsonian primate,[99] STN has been used more commonly in many clinical sites. However, recent studies showed that the stimulation of GPi is equally effective as that of STN.[100,102–105] More details regarding the effect of STN-DBS and GPi-DBS on parkinsonian symptoms are provided in several review articles of DBS.[106–109]

A particular concern regarding STN-DBS and GPi-DBS treatment is the diminishing therapeutic effect on PD motor deficits over time. Although it has been suggested that PIGD is improved by both STN-DBS and GPi-DBS within a year after surgery, recent research has indicated that the effects of basal ganglia stimulation on PIGD may diminish significantly over time. St George and colleagues[110] conducted a metaregression of 12 long-term studies of bilateral STN-DBS and GPi-DBS to investigate the effects of DBS on PIGD and other PD cardinal features (ie, tremor, bradykinesia, and rigidity) based on adjusted UPDRS scores. The data revealed that both STN-DBS and GPi-DBS initially improved PIGD, but these symptoms worsened significantly as time progressed. Similar diminishment of DBS effects was not observed on other cardinal PD features, but immediate postsurgery improvements were maintained. These trends are consistent with the previous studies investigating the long-term effects of DBS on PD motor features.[111–113] These results might indicate that

GPi-DBS and STN-DBS indirectly improve gait initially by directly improving rigidity and bradykinesia. However, over time, these stimulation effects become less prominent as the sensorimotor control underlying postural control and gait worsens with progression of PD.

As levodopa treatment and traditional DBS targeting have been shown to minimally ameliorate PIGD symptoms in persons with PD, recent research on stimulation of the PPN has been introduced with some promising results. Improvements in PIGD, reduction of FOG, and reduced risk of falling have been observed as a result of PPN-DBS (see **Table 2**).[21,22,30–32,114–116] Plaha and Gill[21] first reported the pronounced effect of PPN-DBS on PIGD in both On and Off medication states in 2 persons with PD. This benefit of PPN-DBS in PIGD seemed to be more pronounced than STN-DBS, as shown by the larger clinical change in UPDRS axial subscore (item 27–30) promoted by PPN-DBS.[114] Moreover, Strafella and colleagues[117] recently reported that PPN-DBS increased regional cerebral blood flow in different subcortical structures, particularly the thalamus, and improved the UPDRS motor score in 1 person with PD. Although further studies with larger sample size, involving carefully selected drug-resistant population and inclusion of persons with and without STN or GPi-DBS, are necessary to better understand the benefits of PPN-DBS on PIGD compared with other DBS targets, it seems that PPN-DBS is more effective in improving PIGD in persons with PD than stimulation of the STN and GPi.

Physical Therapy Interventions

In addition to pharmacologic and surgical treatment, short-term therapy-based and exercise interventions may also be effective and feasible options to delay or reverse the progression of PIGD in persons with PD.

The use of extrinsic (visual or auditory) sensory cues has been shown to improve gait in persons with PD.[118–123] Cueing is defined as the application of visual or auditory external stimuli associated with the initiation and ongoing facilitation of gait.[124] When an external cue is given, the gait parameters change constantly to adapt to the changing conditions of the environment. McIntosh and colleagues[119] showed that rhythmical auditory stimulation could positively increase the temporal parameters of gait in persons with PD. Cueing techniques such as musical beats, metronomes, or rhythmical clapping have been implemented as strategies for improving gait for persons with PD.[118,124] Cadence and amplitude are altered when an external auditory cue is present,[119,120] which suggests that repetitive auditory inputs may simply provide a nonspecific arousal stimulus that improves gait function.[121] Visual cues have shown similar effects on the gait patterns of persons with PD.[122,123]

Exercise has also been recommended for persons with PD because of the established relationship between exercise and improved cardiovascular and physical function as well as overall health and well-being.[125,126] There is a large body of empirical evidence that describes the benefits of various exercise interventions (including, but not limited to, progressive resistance training, tai chi [TC] exercise, and aerobic treadmill training) on motor function in persons with PD.

Resistance training in persons with PD has shown robust improvements in physical function and significant lessening of PD motor symptoms (see **Table 2**).[73,74,127] Dibble and colleagues[128] reported that a 12-week high-force eccentric resistance training program significantly improved muscle size and force production of the quadriceps femoris muscle, which was associated with increased scores in strength-related gait tasks (6-minute walk and stair ascend/descend tests) in 10 persons with PD. To further understand how the improvement resulting from resistance training positively affects PIGD in persons with PD, Hass and colleagues[49] recently investigated the effect of 10 weeks of progressive resistance training on GI in persons with PD. They observed more efficient APAs and increases in initial step length and velocity in persons with PD after resistance training. These results were coupled with significant improvements in lower extremity muscle strength. Thus, these findings might suggest the potential of progressive resistance training to reduce PIGD by improving muscle strength in persons with PD, although further investigations with larger sample sizes are needed.

Tai chi (TC) has been also shown to be effective in improving balance and gait in healthy older adults.[129–140] Because of the safe and simple nature of TC training, TC has gained attention as a possible intervention to improve PIGD in persons with PD as well (see **Table 2**). However, research on the effects of TC exercise interventions on PIGD in persons with PD has shown conflicting results.[141–146] Li and colleagues[141] recently reported that gait velocity significantly improved after 24 weeks of TC training. Kim and colleagues[143] also reported a significant improvement in GI performance in persons with PD after participation in a 12-week TC intervention. In contrast, multiple studies have failed to observe any improvements in gait after long-term TC training.[142,145] Most TC studies in PD populations have evaluated motor function using clinical scales such as the Berg Balance Score and UPDRS. Therefore, further studies should implement more objective biomechanical evaluation of motor performance to further investigate the effectiveness of TC on PIGD in persons with PD. Refinement of TC training regimens also seems to be essential for maximizing improvements in PIGD. Thus, future research should focus not only on whether or not TC improves PIGD in persons with PD but also how TC interventions can be designed so that they are optimally effective for persons at various stages of the disease.

Aerobic exercise, particularly chronic treadmill training (TT), has also been suggested to effectively ameliorate parkinsonian locomotor deficits (see **Table 2**). Overground gait has been shown to improve after TT, as shown by increases in stride length and gait speed[147] and step length[148,149] as well as decreases in double-limb support time[150] and stride-to-stride gait variability.[151] Some studies have also suggested that fall incidence[152] and fear of falling[153] were reduced after TT. Post-TT improvement of global parkinsonian disability as evaluated by the UPDRS has also been commonly observed.[147,154,155] There seems to be a mechanism specific to TT that drives the observed gait improvements, extending beyond the cardiovascular and physiologic benefits of generalized aerobic exercise, because overground gait training has not yielded similarly promising results in this population.[150] It has been hypothesized that persons with PD are able to use the proprioceptive feedback from the continuous movement of the treadmill belts to facilitate alterations and improvements in their gait patterns.[148]

Recent research has begun to explore the effectiveness of other forms of TT on locomotion in persons with PD. Previous studies have suggested that body weight–supported TT may induce similar improvements in gait compared with conventional TT in PD.[154,156] Moreover, this type of treadmill exercise may be beneficial to persons at more advanced disease stages who may be unable to tolerate the intensity of repetitive conventional treadmill exercise. Split-belt TT also represents a novel approach to gait rehabilitation in that the walker must adapt and learn a new gait pattern while undergoing aerobic exercise. Although research regarding split-belt TT in PD is still in its infancy, we speculate that some of the improvements in gait symmetry and global gait function observed in persons after stroke[157,158] as a result of these interventions may also substantially benefit persons with PD.

SUMMARY

Persons with PD have motor deficits resulting from dopaminergic dysfunction of the basal ganglia and associated neural pathways. PIGD are particularly debilitating motor features of persons with PD. Parkinsonian gait is characterized by bradykinesia, stooped posture, high stride-to-stride variability, and, in some persons, freezing episodes. Persons with PD also show decreased stability during both static and dynamic motor tasks. These features, among others, contribute to the multifactorial nature of increased fall risk observed in persons with PD. Various pharmacologic, surgical, and exercise-based treatment methods have been suggested to alleviate PIGD symptoms with varying degrees of effectiveness. Although much progress has been made in the evaluation and treatment of PIGD in persons with PD, future research should attempt to further understanding of parkinsonian motor deficits by integrating neurologic, physiologic, and biomechanical perspectives. In addition, researchers should continue to focus both on developing new techniques to address PIGD and on optimizing the therapeutic methods that are currently available.

REFERENCES

1. Horak FB, Nutt JG, Nashner LM. Postural inflexibility in parkinsonian subjects. J Neurol Sci 1992;111(1):46–58.
2. Bloem BR, Hausdorff JM, Visser JE, et al. Falls and freezing of gait in Parkinson's disease: a review of two interconnected, episodic phenomena. Mov Disord 2004;19(8):871–84.
3. Melton LJ, Leibson CL, Achenbach SJ, et al. Fracture risk after the diagnosis of Parkinson's disease: influence of concomitant dementia. Mov Disord 2006; 21(9):1361–7.
4. Johnell O, Melton LJ, Atkinson EJ, et al. Fracture risk in patients with parkinsonism: a population-based study in Olmsted County, Minnesota. Age Ageing 1992;21(1):32–8.
5. Hely MA, Reid WG, Adena MA, et al. The Sydney multicenter study of Parkinson's disease: the inevitability of dementia at 20 years. Mov Disord 2008; 23(6):837–44.
6. Alexander GE, DeLong MR, Strick PL. Parallel organization of functionally segregated circuits linking basal ganglia and cortex. Annu Rev Neurosci 1986;9: 357–81.
7. Kemp JM, Powell TP. The connexions of the striatum and globus pallidus: synthesis and speculation. Philos Trans R Soc Lond B Biol Sci 1971;262(845): 441–57.
8. Evarts EV, Wise SP. Basal ganglia outputs and motor control. Ciba Found Symp 1984;107:83–102.
9. Nambu A, Tokuno H, Takada M. Functional significance of the cortico-subthalamo-pallidal 'hyperdirect' pathway. Neurosci Res 2002;43(2):111–7.
10. Albin RL, Young AB, Penney JB. The functional anatomy of basal ganglia disorders. Trends Neurosci 1989;12(10):366–75.
11. Alexander GE, Crutcher MD. Preparation for movement: neural representations of intended direction in three motor areas of the monkey. J Neurophysiol 1990; 64(1):133–50.
12. Mink JW. The basal ganglia: focused selection and inhibition of competing motor programs. Prog Neurobiol 1996;50(4):381–425.

13. Nambu A, Tokuno H, Hamada I, et al. Excitatory cortical inputs to pallidal neurons via the subthalamic nucleus in the monkey. J Neurophysiol 2000; 84(1):289–300.
14. DeLong MR. Primate models of movement disorders of basal ganglia origin. Trends Neurosci 1990;13(7):281–5.
15. Mink JW, Thach WT. Basal ganglia intrinsic circuits and their role in behavior. Curr Opin Neurobiol 1993;3(6):950–7.
16. Hassler R. Zur Pathologie der Paralysis agitains und des postenzephalitischen Parkinsonismus. J Psychol Neurol 1938;48:387–476.
17. Fearnley JM, Lees AJ. Ageing and Parkinson's disease: substantia nigra regional selectivity. Brain 1991;114(Pt 5):2283–301.
18. Knutsson E. An analysis of parkinsonian gait. Brain 1972;95(3):475–86.
19. Lee MS, Rinne JO, Marsden CD. The pedunculopontine nucleus: its role in the genesis of movement disorders. Yonsei Med J 2000;41(2):167–84.
20. Shute CC, Lewis PR. The ascending cholinergic reticular system: neocortical, olfactory and subcortical projections. Brain 1967;90(3):497–520.
21. Plaha P, Gill SS. Bilateral deep brain stimulation of the pedunculopontine nucleus for Parkinson's disease. Neuroreport 2005;16(17):1883–7.
22. Mazzone P, Lozano A, Stanzione P, et al. Implantation of human pedunculopontine nucleus: a safe and clinically relevant target in Parkinson's disease. Neuroreport 2005;16(17):1877–81.
23. Hirsch EC, Graybiel AM, Duyckaerts C, et al. Neuronal loss in the pedunculopontine tegmental nucleus in Parkinson disease and in progressive supranuclear palsy. Proc Natl Acad Sci U S A 1987;84(16):5976–80.
24. Karachi C, Grabli D, Bernard FA, et al. Cholinergic mesencephalic neurons are involved in gait and postural disorders in Parkinson disease. J Clin Invest 2010; 120(8):2745–54.
25. Yeo SS, Lee DG, Choi BY, et al. Neural connectivity of the pedunculopontine nucleus in relation to walking ability in chronic patients with intracerebral hemorrhage. Eur Neurol 2012;67(4):226–31.
26. Aravamuthan BR, Muthusamy KA, Stein JF, et al. Topography of cortical and subcortical connections of the human pedunculopontine and subthalamic nuclei. Neuroimage 2007;37(3):694–705.
27. Pierantozzi M, Palmieri MG, Galati S, et al. Pedunculopontine nucleus deep brain stimulation changes spinal cord excitability in Parkinson's disease patients. J Neural Transm 2008;115(5):731–5.
28. Schweder PM, Hansen PC, Green AL, et al. Connectivity of the pedunculopontine nucleus in parkinsonian freezing of gait. Neuroreport 2010;21(14):914–6.
29. Lewis SJ, Barker RA. A pathophysiological model of freezing of gait in Parkinson's disease. Parkinsonism Relat Disord 2009;15(5):333–8.
30. Thevathasan W, Coyne TJ, Hyam JA, et al. Pedunculopontine nucleus stimulation improves gait freezing in Parkinson disease. Neurosurgery 2011;69(6): 1248–53 [discussion: 1254].
31. Thevathasan W, Cole MH, Graepel CL, et al. A spatiotemporal analysis of gait freezing and the impact of pedunculopontine nucleus stimulation. Brain 2012; 135(Pt 5):1446–54.
32. Ferraye MU, Debu B, Fraix V, et al. Effects of pedunculopontine nucleus area stimulation on gait disorders in Parkinson's disease. Brain 2010;133(Pt 1):205–14.
33. Wilcox RA, Cole MH, Wong D, et al. Pedunculopontine nucleus deep brain stimulation produces sustained improvement in primary progressive freezing of gait. J Neurol Neurosurg Psychiatry 2011;82(11):1256–9.

34. Wu T, Hallett M. A functional MRI study of automatic movements in patients with Parkinson's disease. Brain 2005;128(Pt 10):2250–9.

35. Yu H, Sternad D, Corcos DM, et al. Role of hyperactive cerebellum and motor cortex in Parkinson's disease. Neuroimage 2007;35(1):222–33.

36. Cerasa A, Hagberg GE, Peppe A, et al. Functional changes in the activity of cerebellum and frontostriatal regions during externally and internally timed movement in Parkinson's disease. Brain Res Bull 2006;71(1–3):259–69.

37. Hanakawa T, Katsumi Y, Fukuyama H, et al. Mechanisms underlying gait disturbance in Parkinson's disease: a single photon emission computed tomography study. Brain 1999;122(Pt 7):1271–82.

38. Jayaram G, Galea JM, Bastian AJ, et al. Human locomotor adaptive learning is proportional to depression of cerebellar excitability. Cereb Cortex 2011;21(8):1901–9.

39. Hausdorff JM. Gait dynamics in Parkinson's disease: common and distinct behavior among stride length, gait variability, and fractal-like scaling. Chaos 2009;19(2):026113.

40. Hely MA, Morris JG, Traficante R, et al. The Sydney Multicentre Study of Parkinson's Disease: progression and mortality at 10 years. J Neurol Neurosurg Psychiatry 1999;67(3):300–7.

41. Fahn S. Does levodopa slow or hasten the rate of progression of Parkinson's disease? J Neurol 2005;252(Suppl 4):IV37–42.

42. Morris ME, Huxham F, McGinley J, et al. The biomechanics and motor control of gait in Parkinson disease. Clin Biomech (Bristol, Avon) 2001;16(6):459–70.

43. Roemmich RT, Nocera JR, Vallabhajosula S, et al. Spatiotemporal variability during gait initiation in Parkinson's disease. Gait Posture 2012;36:340–3.

44. Lewek MD, Poole R, Johnson J, et al. Arm swing magnitude and asymmetry during gait in the early stages of Parkinson's disease. Gait Posture 2010;31(2):256–60.

45. Morris ME, Iansek R, Matyas TA, et al. The pathogenesis of gait hypokinesia in Parkinson's disease. Brain 1994;117(Pt 5):1169–81.

46. Morris ME, Iansek R, Matyas TA, et al. Stride length regulation in Parkinson's disease. Normalization strategies and underlying mechanisms. Brain 1996;119(Pt 2):551–68.

47. Gray P, Hildebrand K. Fall risk factors in Parkinson's disease. J Neurosci Nurs 2000;32(4):222–8.

48. Stack E, Ashburn A. Fall events described by people with Parkinson's disease: implications for clinical interviewing and the research agenda. Physiother Res Int 1999;4(3):190–200.

49. Hass CJ, Buckley TA, Pitsikoulis C, et al. Progressive resistance training improves gait initiation in individuals with Parkinson's disease. Gait Posture 2012;35(4):669–73.

50. Halliday SE, Winter DA, Frank JS, et al. The initiation of gait in young, elderly, and Parkinson's disease subjects. Gait Posture 1998;8(1):8–14.

51. Hass CJ, Waddell DE, Fleming RP, et al. Gait initiation and dynamic balance control in Parkinson's disease. Arch Phys Med Rehabil 2005;86(11):2172–6.

52. Bishop M, Brunt D, Marjama-Lyons J. Do people with Parkinson's disease change strategy during unplanned gait termination? Neurosci Lett 2006;397(3):240–4.

53. Martin M, Shinberg M, Kuchibhatla M, et al. Gait initiation in community-dwelling adults with Parkinson disease: comparison with older and younger adults without the disease. Phys Ther 2002;82(6):566–77.

54. Schaafsma JD, Balash Y, Gurevich T, et al. Characterization of freezing of gait subtypes and the response of each to levodopa in Parkinson's disease. Eur J Neurol 2003;10(4):391–8.

55. Winter DA, Patla AE, Frank JS. Assessment of balance control in humans. Med Prog Technol 1990;16(1–2):31–51.

56. Chang H, Krebs DE. Dynamic balance control in elders: gait initiation assessment as a screening tool. Arch Phys Med Rehabil 1999;80(5):490–4.

57. Cutsuridis V. Origins of a repetitive and co-contractive biphasic pattern of muscle activation in Parkinson's disease. Neural Netw 2011;24(6):592–601.

58. Miller RA, Thaut MH, McIntosh GC, et al. Components of EMG symmetry and variability in parkinsonian and healthy elderly gait. Electroencephalogr Clin Neurophysiol 1996;101(1):1–7.

59. Pfann KD, Buchman AS, Comella CL, et al. Control of movement distance in Parkinson's disease. Mov Disord 2001;16(6):1048–65.

60. Salenius S, Avikainen S, Kaakkola S, et al. Defective cortical drive to muscle in Parkinson's disease and its improvement with levodopa. Brain 2002;125(Pt 3): 491–500.

61. Dalton E, Bishop M, Tillman MD, et al. Simple change in initial standing position enhances the initiation of gait. Med Sci Sports Exerc 2011;43(12):2352–8.

62. O'Sullivan JD, Said CM, Dillon LC, et al. Gait analysis in patients with Parkinson's disease and motor fluctuations: influence of levodopa and comparison with other measures of motor function. Mov Disord 1998;13(6):900–6.

63. Ashburn A, Stack E, Pickering RM, et al. A community-dwelling sample of people with Parkinson's disease: characteristics of fallers and non-fallers. Age Ageing 2001;30(1):47–52.

64. Cole MH, Silburn PA, Wood JM, et al. Falls in Parkinson's disease: evidence for altered stepping strategies on compliant surfaces. Parkinsonism Relat Disord 2011;17(8):610–6.

65. Giladi N, Shabtai H, Rozenberg E, et al. Gait festination in Parkinson's disease. Parkinsonism Relat Disord 2001;7(2):135–8.

66. Plotnik M, Hausdorff JM. The role of gait rhythmicity and bilateral coordination of stepping in the pathophysiology of freezing of gait in Parkinson's disease. Mov Disord 2008;23(S2):S444–50.

67. Yogev G, Giladi N, Peretz C, et al. Dual tasking, gait rhythmicity, and Parkinson's disease: which aspects of gait are attention demanding? Eur J Neurosci 2005; 22(5):1248–56.

68. Mbourou GA, Lajoie Y, Teasdale N. Step length variability at gait initiation in elderly fallers and non-fallers, and young adults. Gerontology 2003;49(1): 21–6.

69. Brach JS, Berlin JE, VanSwearingen JM, et al. Too much or too little step width variability is associated with a fall history in older persons who walk at or near normal gait speed. J Neuroeng Rehabil 2005;2:21.

70. Barak Y, Wagenaar RC, Holt KG. Gait characteristics of elderly people with a history of falls: a dynamic approach. Phys Ther 2006;86(11):1501–10.

71. Hase K, Stein RB. Analysis of rapid stopping during human walking. J Neurophysiol 1998;80(1):255–61.

72. Stelmach GE, Teasdale N, Phillips J, et al. Force production characteristics in Parkinson's disease. Exp Brain Res 1989;76(1):165–72.

73. Corcos DM, Chen CM, Quinn NP, et al. Strength in Parkinson's disease: relationship to rate of force generation and clinical status. Ann Neurol 1996;39(1): 79–88.

74. David FJ, Rafferty MR, Robichaud JA, et al. Progressive resistance exercise and Parkinson's disease: a review of potential mechanisms. Parkinsons Dis 2012; 2012:124527.
75. Robichaud JA, Pfann KD, Comella CL, et al. Effect of medication on EMG patterns in individuals with Parkinson's disease. Mov Disord 2002;17(5):950–60.
76. Bishop MD, Brunt D, Pathare N, et al. The interaction between leading and trailing limbs during stopping in humans. Neurosci Lett 2002;323(1):1–4.
77. Crenna P, Cuong DM, Breniere Y. Motor programmes for the termination of gait in humans: organisation and velocity-dependent adaptation. J Physiol 2001; 537(Pt 3):1059–72.
78. Rubenstein LZ. Falls in older people: epidemiology, risk factors and strategies for prevention. Age Ageing 2006;35(Suppl 2):ii37–41.
79. Bloem BR, Grimbergen YA, Cramer M, et al. Prospective assessment of falls in Parkinson's disease. J Neurol 2001;248(11):950–8.
80. Bloem BR, van Vugt JP, Beckley DJ. Postural instability and falls in Parkinson's disease. Adv Neurol 2001;87:209–23.
81. Morris ME, Huxham FE, McGinley J, et al. Gait disorders and gait rehabilitation in Parkinson's disease. Adv Neurol 2001;87:347–61.
82. Kerr GK, Worringham CJ, Cole MH, et al. Predictors of future falls in Parkinson disease. Neurology 2010;75(2):116–24.
83. Lamberti P, Armenise S, Castaldo V, et al. Freezing gait in Parkinson's disease. Eur Neurol 1997;38(4):297–301.
84. Nutt JG, Bloem BR, Giladi N, et al. Freezing of gait: moving forward on a mysterious clinical phenomenon. Lancet Neurol 2011;10(8):734–44.
85. Lee SJ, Yoo JY, Ryu JS, et al. The effects of visual and auditory cues on freezing of gait in patients with Parkinson disease. Am J Phys Med Rehabil 2012;91(1): 2–11.
86. Stewart KC, Fernandez HH, Okun MS, et al. Distribution of motor impairment influences quality of life in Parkinson's disease. Mov Disord 2008;23(10): 1466–8.
87. Rahman S, Griffin HJ, Quinn NP, et al. Quality of life in Parkinson's disease: the relative importance of the symptoms. Mov Disord 2008;23(10):1428–34.
88. Chapuis S, Ouchchane L, Metz O, et al. Impact of the motor complications of Parkinson's disease on the quality of life. Mov Disord 2005;20(2):224–30.
89. Chen R. Paradoxical worsening of gait with levodopa in Parkinson disease. Neurology 2012;78(7):446–7.
90. Vokaer M, Azar NA, de Beyl DZ. Effects of levodopa on upper limb mobility and gait in Parkinson's disease. J Neurol Neurosurg Psychiatry 2003;74(9):1304–7.
91. Blin O, Ferrandez AM, Pailhous J, et al. Dopa-sensitive and dopa-resistant gait parameters in Parkinson's disease. J Neurol Sci 1991;103(1):51–4.
92. Devos D, Defebvre L, Bordet R. Dopaminergic and non-dopaminergic pharmacological hypotheses for gait disorders in Parkinson's disease. Fundam Clin Pharmacol 2010;24(4):407–21.
93. Espay AJ, Fasano A, van Nuenen BF, et al. "On" state freezing of gait in Parkinson disease: a paradoxical levodopa-induced complication. Neurology 2012; 78(7):454–7.
94. Olanow CW, Brin MF, Obeso JA. The role of deep brain stimulation as a surgical treatment for Parkinson's disease. Neurology 2000;55(12 Suppl 6):S60–6.
95. Kumar R, Lozano AM, Kim YJ, et al. Double-blind evaluation of subthalamic nucleus deep brain stimulation in advanced Parkinson's disease. Neurology 1998;51(3):850–5.

96. Wichmann T, Bergman H, DeLong MR. The primate subthalamic nucleus. III. Changes in motor behavior and neuronal activity in the internal pallidum induced by subthalamic inactivation in the MPTP model of parkinsonism. J Neurophysiol 1994;72(2):521–30.

97. Lozano AM, Lang AE, Galvez-Jimenez N, et al. Effect of GPi pallidotomy on motor function in Parkinson's disease. Lancet 1995;346(8987):1383–7.

98. Aziz TZ, Peggs D, Sambrook MA, et al. Lesion of the subthalamic nucleus for the alleviation of 1-methyl-4-phenyl-1,2,3,6-tetrahydropyridine (MPTP)-induced parkinsonism in the primate. Mov Disord 1991;6(4):288–92.

99. Bergman H, Wichmann T, DeLong MR. Reversal of experimental parkinsonism by lesions of the subthalamic nucleus. Science 1990;249(4975):1436–8.

100. Follett KA, Weaver FM, Stern M, et al. Pallidal versus subthalamic deep-brain stimulation for Parkinson's disease. N Engl J Med 2010;362(22):2077–91.

101. Benabid AL, Chabardes S, Mitrofanis J, et al. Deep brain stimulation of the subthalamic nucleus for the treatment of Parkinson's disease. Lancet Neurol 2009;8(1):67–81.

102. Follett KA, Torres-Russotto D. Deep brain stimulation of globus pallidus interna, subthalamic nucleus, and pedunculopontine nucleus for Parkinson's disease: which target? Parkinsonism Relat Disord 2012;18(Suppl 1):S165–7.

103. Limousin P, Martinez-Torres I. Deep brain stimulation for Parkinson's disease. Neurotherapeutics 2008;5(2):309–19.

104. Okun MS, Foote KD. Subthalamic nucleus vs globus pallidus interna deep brain stimulation, the rematch: will pallidal deep brain stimulation make a triumphant return? Arch Neurol 2005;62(4):533–6.

105. Okun MS, Fernandez HH, Wu SS, et al. Cognition and mood in Parkinson's disease in subthalamic nucleus versus globus pallidus interna deep brain stimulation: the COMPARE trial. Ann Neurol 2009;65(5):586–95.

106. Bronstein JM, Tagliati M, Alterman RL, et al. Deep brain stimulation for Parkinson disease: an expert consensus and review of key issues. Arch Neurol 2011;68(2):165.

107. Weaver F, Follett K, Hur K, et al. Deep brain stimulation in Parkinson disease: a metaanalysis of patient outcomes. J Neurosurg 2005;103(6):956–67.

108. Fasano A, Daniele A, Albanese A. Treatment of motor and non-motor features of Parkinson's disease with deep brain stimulation. Lancet Neurol 2012;11(5):429–42.

109. Okun MS, Foote KD. Parkinson's disease DBS: what, when, who and why? The time has come to tailor DBS targets. Expert Rev Neurother 2010;10(12):1847–57.

110. St George RJ, Nutt JG, Burchiel KJ, et al. A meta-regression of the long-term effects of deep brain stimulation on balance and gait in PD. Neurology 2010;75(14):1292–9.

111. Rodriguez-Oroz MC, Obeso JA, Lang AE, et al. Bilateral deep brain stimulation in Parkinson's disease: a multicentre study with 4 years follow-up. Brain 2005;128(Pt 10):2240–9.

112. Gan J, Xie-Brustolin J, Mertens P, et al. Bilateral subthalamic nucleus stimulation in advanced Parkinson's disease: three years follow-up. J Neurol 2007;254(1):99–106.

113. Ostergaard K, Aa Sunde N. Evolution of Parkinson's disease during 4 years of bilateral deep brain stimulation of the subthalamic nucleus. Mov Disord 2006;21(5):624–31.

114. Stefani A, Lozano AM, Peppe A, et al. Bilateral deep brain stimulation of the pedunculopontine and subthalamic nuclei in severe Parkinson's disease. Brain 2007;130(Pt 6):1596–607.

115. Moro E, Hamani C, Poon YY, et al. Unilateral pedunculopontine stimulation improves falls in Parkinson's disease. Brain 2010;133(Pt 1):215–24.

116. Lozano AM. Deep brain stimulation for Parkinson disease. J Neurosurg 2010; 112(3):477 [discussion: 477–8].

117. Strafella AP, Lozano AM, Ballanger B, et al. rCBF changes associated with PPN stimulation in a patient with Parkinson's disease: a PET study. Mov Disord 2008; 23(7):1051–4.

118. Suteerawattananon M, Morris GS, Etnyre BR, et al. Effects of visual and auditory cues on gait in individuals with Parkinson's disease. J Neurol Sci 2004;219(1–2): 63–9.

119. McIntosh GC, Brown SH, Rice RR, et al. Rhythmic auditory-motor facilitation of gait patterns in patients with Parkinson's disease. J Neurol Neurosurg Psychiatry 1997;62(1):22–6.

120. Ford MP, Malone LA, Nyikos I, et al. Gait training with progressive external auditory cueing in persons with Parkinson's disease. Arch Phys Med Rehabil 2010; 91(8):1255–61.

121. Howe TE, Lovgreen B, Cody FW, et al. Auditory cues can modify the gait of persons with early-stage Parkinson's disease: a method for enhancing parkinsonian walking performance? Clin Rehabil 2003;17(4):363–7.

122. Dunne JW, Hankey GJ, Edis RH. Parkinsonism: upturned walking stick as an aid to locomotion. Arch Phys Med Rehabil 1987;68(6):380–1.

123. Bagley S, Kelly B, Tunnicliffe N, et al. The effect of visual cues on the gait of independently mobile Parkinson's disease patients. Physiotherapy 1991;77(6): 415–20.

124. Nieuwboer A, Kwakkel G, Rochester L, et al. Cueing training in the home improves gait-related mobility in Parkinson's disease: the RESCUE trial. J Neurol Neurosurg Psychiatry 2007;78(2):134–40.

125. Goodwin VA, Richards SH, Taylor RS, et al. The effectiveness of exercise interventions for people with Parkinson's disease: a systematic review and meta-analysis. Mov Disord 2008;23(5):631–40.

126. Crizzle AM, Newhouse IJ. Is physical exercise beneficial for persons with Parkinson's disease? Clin J Sport Med 2006;16(5):422–5. http://dx.doi.org/ 10.1097/01.jsm.0000244612.55550.7d.

127. Ridgel AL, Kim CH, Fickes EJ, et al. Changes in executive function after acute bouts of passive cycling in Parkinson's disease. J Aging Phys Act 2011;19(2): 87–98.

128. Dibble LE, Hale TF, Marcus RL, et al. High-intensity resistance training amplifies muscle hypertrophy and functional gains in persons with Parkinson's disease. Mov Disord 2006;21(9):1444–52.

129. Li F, Harmer P, Fisher KJ, et al. Tai chi: improving functional balance and predicting subsequent falls in older persons. Med Sci Sports Exerc 2004;36(12): 2046–52.

130. Li F, Harmer P, Fisher KJ, et al. Tai chi and fall reductions in older adults: a randomized controlled trial. J Gerontol A Biol Sci Med Sci 2005;60(2): 187–94.

131. Taggart HM. Effects of tai chi exercise on balance, functional mobility, and fear of falling among older women. Appl Nurs Res 2002;15(4):235–42.

132. Wolf SL, Barnhart HX, Ellison GL, et al. The effect of tai chi quan and computerized balance training on postural stability in older subjects. Atlanta FICSIT Group. Frailty and injuries: cooperative studies on intervention techniques. Phys Ther 1997;77(4):371–81 [discussion: 382–4].

133. Wolf SL, Barnhart HX, Kutner NG, et al. Reducing frailty and falls in older persons: an investigation of tai chi and computerized balance training. Atlanta FICSIT Group. Frailty and injuries: cooperative studies of intervention techniques. J Am Geriatr Soc 1996;44(5):489–97.

134. Wolfson L, Whipple R, Derby C, et al. Balance and strength training in older adults: intervention gains and tai chi maintenance. J Am Geriatr Soc 1996; 44(5):498–506.

135. Wong AM, Lin YC, Chou SW, et al. Coordination exercise and postural stability in elderly people: effect of tai chi chuan. Arch Phys Med Rehabil 2001;82(5): 608–12.

136. Wu G, Zhao F, Zhou X, et al. Improvement of isokinetic knee extensor strength and reduction of postural sway in the elderly from long-term tai chi exercise. Arch Phys Med Rehabil 2002;83(10):1364–9.

137. Taylor-Piliae RE, Newell KA, Cherin R, et al. Effects of tai chi and Western exercise on physical and cognitive functioning in healthy community-dwelling older adults. J Aging Phys Act 2010;18(3):261–79.

138. Song R, Lee EO, Lam P, et al. Effects of tai chi exercise on pain, balance, muscle strength, and perceived difficulties in physical functioning in older women with osteoarthritis: a randomized clinical trial. J Rheumatol 2003;30(9): 2039–44.

139. Lin MR, Hwang HF, Wang YW, et al. Community-based tai chi and its effect on injurious falls, balance, gait, and fear of falling in older people. Phys Ther 2006; 86(9):1189–201.

140. Hass CJ, Gregor RJ, Waddell DE, et al. The influence of tai chi training on the center of pressure trajectory during gait initiation in older adults. Arch Phys Med Rehabil 2004;85(10):1593–8.

141. Li F, Harmer P, Fitzgerald K, et al. Tai chi and postural stability in patients with Parkinson's disease. N Engl J Med 2012;366(6):511–9.

142. Hackney ME, Earhart GM. Tai chi improves balance and mobility in people with Parkinson disease. Gait Posture 2008;28(3):456–60.

143. Kim HD, Kim TY, Jae HD, et al. The effects of tai chi based exercise on dynamic postural control of Parkinson's disease patients while initiating gait. J Phys Ther Sci 2011;23(2):265–9.

144. Klein PJ, Rivers L. Taiji for Individuals with Parkinson disease and their support partners: program evaluation. J Neurol Phys Ther 2006;30(1):22–7. http: //dx.doi.org/10.1097/01.NPT.0000282146.18446.f1.

145. Lee MS, Lam P, Ernst E. Effectiveness of tai chi for Parkinson's disease: a critical review. Parkinsonism Relat Disord 2008;14(8):589–94.

146. Venglar M. Case report: tai chi and parkinsonism. Physiother Res Int 2005;10(2): 116–21.

147. Herman T, Giladi N, Gruendlinger L, et al. Six weeks of intensive treadmill training improves gait and quality of life in patients with Parkinson's disease: a pilot study. Arch Phys Med Rehabil 2007;88(9):1154–8.

148. Bello O, Marquez G, Camblor M, et al. Mechanisms involved in treadmill walking improvements in Parkinson's disease. Gait Posture 2010;32(1):118–23.

149. Bello O, Sanchez JA, Fernandez-del-Olmo M. Treadmill walking in Parkinson's disease patients: adaptation and generalization effect. Mov Disord 2008; 23(9):1243–9.

150. Pohl M, Rockstroh G, Ruckriem S, et al. Immediate effects of speed-dependent treadmill training on gait parameters in early Parkinson's disease. Arch Phys Med Rehabil 2003;84(12):1760–6.

151. Frenkel-Toledo S, Giladi N, Peretz C, et al. Treadmill walking as an external pacemaker to improve gait rhythm and stability in Parkinson's disease. Mov Disord 2005;20(9):1109–14.
152. Protas EJ, Mitchell K, Williams A, et al. Gait and step training to reduce falls in Parkinson's disease. NeuroRehabilitation 2005;20(3):183–90.
153. Cakit BD, Saracoglu M, Genc H, et al. The effects of incremental speed-dependent treadmill training on postural instability and fear of falling in Parkinson's disease. Clin Rehabil 2007;21(8):698–705.
154. Miyai I, Fujimoto Y, Ueda Y, et al. Treadmill training with body weight support: its effect on Parkinson's disease. Arch Phys Med Rehabil 2000;81(7):849–52.
155. Skidmore FM, Patterson SL, Shulman LM, et al. Pilot safety and feasibility study of treadmill aerobic exercise in Parkinson disease with gait impairment. J Rehabil Res Dev 2008;45(1):117–24.
156. Fisher BE, Wu AD, Salem GJ, et al. The effect of exercise training in improving motor performance and corticomotor excitability in people with early Parkinson's disease. Arch Phys Med Rehabil 2008;89(7):1221–9.
157. Reisman DS, Bastian AJ, Morton SM. Neurophysiologic and rehabilitation insights from the split-belt and other locomotor adaptation paradigms. Phys Ther 2010;90(2):187–95.
158. Reisman DS, Wityk R, Silver K, et al. Split-belt treadmill adaptation transfers to overground walking in persons poststroke. Neurorehabil Neural Repair 2009; 23(7):735–44.

Index

Note: Page numbers of article titles are in **boldface** type.

Phys Med Rehabil Clin N Am 24 (2013) 393–401
http://dx.doi.org/10.1016/S1047-9651(13)00009-0
1047-9651/13/$ – see front matter © 2013 Elsevier Inc. All rights reserved.

Moving?

Make sure your subscription moves with you!

To notify us of your new address, find your **Clinics Account Number** (located on your mailing label above your name), and contact customer service at:

Email: journalscustomerservice-usa@elsevier.com

800-654-2452 (subscribers in the U.S. & Canada)
314-447-8871 (subscribers outside of the U.S. & Canada)

Fax number: 314-447-8029

Elsevier Health Sciences Division
Subscription Customer Service
3251 Riverport Lane
Maryland Heights, MO 63043

*To ensure uninterrupted delivery of your subscription, please notify us at least 4 weeks in advance of move.

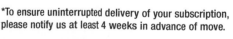

Printed and bound by CPI Group (UK) Ltd, Croydon, CR0 4YY

03/10/2024

01040441-0017